Neuroscience at a Glance

This edition is dedicated to Imogen Rose Barker who died tragically February 2007: a wonderful daughter and an inspiration to many.

Neuroscience at a Glance

Roger A. Barker

BA, MBBS, MRCP, PhD
Cambridge Centre for Brain Repair and Department of Neurology
University of Cambridge
Robinson Way
Cambridge

Stephen Barasi

BSc, PhD
School of Bioscience
Cardiff University
Museum Avenue
Cardiff

and Neuropharmacology by

Michael J. Neal

DSc, PhD, MA, BPharm
Emeritus Professor of Pharmacology
Department of Pharmacology
Kings College
London

Third edition

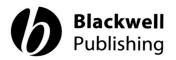

Blackwell Publishing

Published by Blackwell Publishing
Blackwell Publishing, Inc., 350 Main Street, Malden, Massachusetts 02148-5020, USA
Blackwell Publishing Ltd, 9600 Garsington Road, Oxford OX4 2DQ, UK
Blackwell Publishing Asia Pty Ltd, 550 Swanston Street, Carlton, Victoria 3053, Australia

First published 1999
Second edition 2003
Third edition 2008

1   2008

Library of Congress Cataloging-in-Publication Data

Barker, Roger A., 1961–
    Neuroscience at a glance / Roger A. Barker, Stephen Barasi; and neuropharmacology by
Michael J. Neal. – 3rd ed.
        p.   ;   cm.
    ISBN 978-1-4051-5045-3 (alk. paper)
    1. Neurosciences.   I. Barasi, Stephen.   II. Neal, M. J.   III. Title.
    [DNLM: 1. Nervous System Physiology.   2. Nervous System Diseases.   WL 102 B2557n 2008]
    RC341.B326 2008
    612.8–dc22
                                                                            2007025765

A catalogue record for this title is available from the British Library

Set in 9/11.5 pt Times by SNP Best-set Typesetter Ltd., Hong Kong
Printed and bound in Singapore by Markono Print Media Ptd Ltd

Commissioning Editor: Martin Sugden/Vicki Noyes
Development Editor: Karen Moore
Production Controller: Debbie Wyer
Website produced by: Meg Barton and Oliver Brummell

For further information on Blackwell Publishing, visit our website:
http://www.blackwellpublishing.com

The publisher's policy is to use permanent paper from mills that operate a sustainable forestry policy,
and which has been manufactured from pulp processed using acid-free and elementary chlorine-free
practices. Furthermore, the publisher ensures that the text paper and cover board used have met acceptable
environmental accreditation standards.

Contents

Companion website: www.medicalneuroscience.com

Introduction

Neuroscience at a Glance is designed primarily for undergraduate medical students as a revision text or review of basic neuroscience mechanisms, rather than a comprehensive account of the field of medical neuroscience. The book does not attempt to provide a systematic review of clinical neurology. However, it should also be of use for those in clinical training and practice wanting a review and synopsis of the science behind the clinical practice.

The changing nature of medical training in this country has meant that rather than teaching being discipline based (anatomy, physiology, pharmacology, etc.), the current approach is much more integrated with the focus on the entire system. Students pursuing a problem-based learning course will also benefit from the concise presentation of integrated material.

This book summarizes the rapidly expanding field of neuroscience with reference to clinical disorders, such that the material is set in a clinical context. In general, the later chapters contain more clinical material while the earlier ones contain a section towards the end outlining applied neuroscience. However, learning about the organization of the nervous system purely from clinical disorders is short-sighted as the changing nature of medical neuroscience means that areas with little clinical relevance today may become more of an issue in the future. An example of this is ion channels and the recent burgeoning of a host of channelopathies. For this reason some chapters focus more on scientific mechanisms with less clinical emphasis.

Each chapter presents the bulk of its information in the form of an annotated figure, which is expanded in the accompanying text. It is recommended that the figure is worked through with the text rather than just viewed in isolation. The condensed nature of each chapter means that much of the information has to be given in a didactic fashion, but a list of suggested further reading for each chapter is given on the companion website (see below). Although the text focuses on core material, some additional important detail is also included.

The book has broadly been divided up into sections on the structure and biophysics of the nervous system (Chapters 1–19); the sensory components of the nervous system (Chapters 20–33); the motor components of the nervous system (Chapters 34–43); the autonomic, limbic and brainstem systems underlying wakefulness and sleep along with neural plasticity (Chapters 44–50) and, finally, a section on the approach, investigation and range of clinical disorders of the nervous system (Chapters 51–60). A list of further reading and glossaries of neurological conditions and neuroscientific terms are available free of charge from the companion website.

Each section builds on the previous ones to some extent, and so reading the introductory chapter may give a greater understanding to later chapters in that section; for example, the somatosensory system chapter may be better read after the chapter on the general organization of sensory systems.

Companion website

A companion website for this edition of *Neuroscience at a Glance* is available at:

www.medicalneuroscience.com

The website includes the following resources for students:
- Interactive self-assessment multiple-choice questions
- A database of extra case studies
- Further reading lists
- Glossaries of terms
- A forum for your feedback

Acknowledgements

In this the latest edition of the book we have attempted to further integrate the clinical relevance of neurobiology into the text and website. This we have done by including several new chapters of neuropsychiatry and neuropsychology as well as imaging and the introduction of case studies based on real clinical scenarios. We have been very fortunate to recruit the help of Dr Paul Fletcher (Wellcome Senior Fellow and Honorary Consultant Psychiatrist) for the neuropsychiatry/neuropsychology and Dr Justin Cross (Consultant Neuroradiologist) for the imaging. I have provided all the clinical cases, which are based on patients that I have seen over the years.

Finally, I would like to thank all the students that I have taught over the years who have helped me to refine this book as well as Karen Moore and Martin Sugden from Blackwell Publishing for all their help and innovative ideas in this new, more colourful edition of the book.

Roger Barker
Cambridge

List of abbreviations

5-HIAA	5-hydroxy indole acetic acid
5-HT	5-hydroxytryptamine (serotonin)
A1	primary auditory cortex
ACA	anterior cerebral artery
ACh	acetylcholine
AChE	acetylcholinesterase
AChR	acetylcholine receptor
ACTH	adenocorticotrophic hormone
ADH	antidiuretic hormone (vasopressin)
AICA	anterior inferior cerebellar artery
ALS	amyotrophic lateral sclerosis
AMPA-R	α amino-3-hydroxy-5-methyl-4-isoxazole proprionic acid glutamate receptor
ANS	autonomic nervous system
APP	amyloid precursor protein
ATP	adenosine triphosphate
AuD	autosomal dominant
AuR	autosomal recessive
BBB	blood–brain barrier
BM	basilar membrane
BMP	bone morphogenic protein
cAMP	cyclic adenosine monophosphate
CBM	cerebellum
CBP	calcium-binding protein
CCK	cholecystokinin
cf	climbing fibre
cGMP	cyclic guanosine monophosphate
CMCT	central motor conduction time
CMUA	continuous motor unit activity
CNS	central nervous system
CNTF	ciliary neurotrophic factor
COMT	catecholamine-O-methyltransferase
CoST	corticospinal tract
COX	cyclo-oxygenase
CPG	central pattern generator
CPK	creatine phosphokinase
CRH	corticotrophin-releasing hormone
CRPS	complex regional pain syndrome
CSF	cerebrospinal fluid
CT	computerized tomography
CVA	cerebrovascular accident
DA	dopamine
DAG	diacylglycerol
DAT	dementia of the Alzheimer type
dB	decibel
DC	dorsal column
DCN	dorsal column nuclei
DCNN	deep cerebellar nuclei neurone
DMD	Duchenne's muscular dystrophy
DNA	deoxyribonucleic acid
DRG	dorsal root ganglia
DSCT	dorsal spinocerebellar tract
DSIP	delta sleep-inducing peptide
ECG	electrocardiography/electrocardiogram
ECT	electroconvulsive therapy
EEG	electroencephalography/electroencephalogram
EMG	electromyography/electromyogram
enk	enkephalin
EP	evoked potential
epp	end-plate potential
EPSP	excitatory postsynaptic potential
FEF	frontal eye field
fMRI	functional magnetic resonance imaging
FTD	frontotemporal dementia
GABA	γ-aminobutyric acid
GABA-R	γ-aminobutyric acid receptor
GAD	glutamic acid decarboxylase
GDNF	glial cell line derived neurotrophic factor
Glut-R	glutamate receptor
GoC	Golgi cell
G$_{olf}$	G-protein associated with olfactory receptors
GPe	globus pallidus external segment
GPi	globus pallidus internal segment
G-protein	guanosine triphosphate-binding protein
GrC	granule cell
GTO	Golgi tendon organ
GTP	guanosine triphosphate
HLA	histocompatibility locus antigen
HMM	heavy meromyosin
HMSN	hereditary motor sensory neuropathy
HTM	high-threshold mechanoreceptor
Hz	hertz
IC	inferior colliculus
ICA	internal carotid artery
IHC	inner hair cell
IL	intralaminar nuclei of the thalamus
IN	interneurone
IP$_3$	inositol triphosphate
IPSP	inhibitory postsynaptic potential
JPS	joint position sense
LEMS	Lambert–Eaton myasthenic syndrome
LGMD	limb girdle muscular dystrophy
LGN	lateral geniculate nucleus of the thalamus
LMM	light meromyosin
LMN	lower motorneurone
LTD	long-term depression
LTP	long-term potentiation
MAO	monoamine oxidase
MAO$_A$	monoamine oxidase type A
MAO$_B$	monoamine oxidase type B
MAOI	monoamine oxidase inhibitor
MCA	middle cerebral artery
MCS	minimally conscious state
MD	mediodorsal nucleus of the thalamus
mepp	miniature end-plate potential
MGN	medial geniculate nucleus of the thalamus
MHC	major histocompatibility complex
MLF	medial longitudinal fasciculus
MN	motorneurone
MND	motorneurone disease

MRA	magnetic resonance angiography	**SA**	slowly adapting receptor
MRI	magentic resonance imaging	**SCA**	spinocerebellar ataxia
MRV	magnetic resonance venography	**SMA**	supplementary motor area
MsI	primary motor cortex	**SmI**	primary somatosensory cortex
MUSK	muscle specific kinase	**SmII**	secondary somatosensory area
NA	noradrenaline (norepinephrine)	**SNAP**	soluble NSF attachment protein
NCS	nerve conduction studies	**SNARE**	SNAP receptor
NFT	neurofibrillary tangle	**SNc**	substantia nigra pars compacta
NGF	nerve growth factor	**SNP**	senile neuritic plaques
NMDA	N-methyl-D-aspartate	**SNr**	substantia nigra pars reticulata
NMDA-R	N-methyl-D aspartate glutamate receptor	**SNS**	sympathetic nervous system
NMJ	neuromuscular junction	**SOC**	superior olivary complex
NO	nitric oxide	**SP**	substance P
NS	neostriatum	**SPECT**	single photon emission computed tomography
NSAID	non-steroidal anti-inflammatory drug	**SR**	sarcoplasmic reticulum
OD	ocular dominance	**SSRI**	selective serotonin reuptake inhibitor
OHC	outer hair cell	**STN**	subthalamic nucleus
PAG	periaqueductal grey matter	**STT**	spinothalamic tract
PCA	posterior cerebral artery	**SVZ**	subventricular zone
PDE	phosphodiesterase	**SWS**	slow-wave sleep
PET	positron emission tomography	**TENS**	transcutaneous nerve stimulation
pf	parallel fibre	**TeST**	tectospinal tract
PG	prostaglandin	**TIA**	transient ischaemic attack
PGO	pontine–geniculo-occipital	**TM**	tectorial membrane
PICA	posterior inferior cerebellar artery	**TNF**	tumour necrosis factor
PMC	premotor cortex	**TRH**	thyrotrophin-releasing hormone
PMN	polymodal nociceptors	**T-tubule**	transverse tubule
PMP	peripheral myelin protein	**UMN**	upper motorneurone
PNS	peripheral nervous system	**UPS**	ubiquitin–proteosome system
PPC	posterior parietal cortex	**V1**	primary visual cortex (Brodmann's area 17)
PPN	pedunculopontine nucleus	**VA–VL**	ventroanterior–ventrolateral nuclei of the thalamus
PPRF	paramedian pontine reticular formation	**VCN**	ventral cochlear nucleus
PuC	Purkinje cell	**VEP**	visual evoked potential
RA	rapidly adapting receptor	**VeST**	vestibulospinal tract
REM	rapid eye movement	**VLPA**	ventrolateral preoptic area
ReST	reticulospinal tract	**VOR**	vestibulo-ocular reflex
RiMLF	rostral interstitial nucleus of the medial longitudinal fasciculus	**VP**	ventroposterior nucleus of the thalamus
RMS	rostral migratory stream	**VPL**	ventroposterior nucleus of the thalamus, lateral part
RN	raphe nucleus	**VPM**	ventroposterior nucleus of the thalamus, medial part
RNA	ribonucleic acid	**VPT**	vibration perception threshold
RuST	rubrospinal tract	**VSCT**	ventral spinocerebellar tract

1 The organization of the nervous system

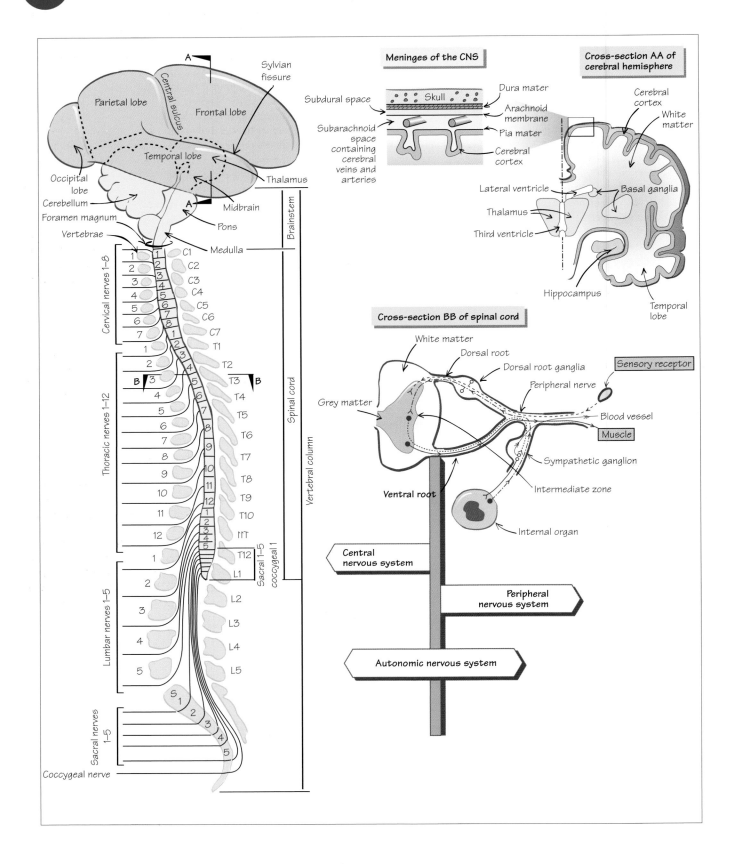

An overview

The nervous system can be divided into three major parts: the **peripheral** (PNS), **central** (CNS) and **autonomic** (ANS) **nervous system**. The PNS is defined as those nerves that lie outside the brain, brainstem or spinal cord, while the CNS embraces those cells that lie within these structures.

Peripheral nervous system

The PNS consists of nerve trunks made up of both afferent fibres or axons conducting sensory information to the spinal cord and brainstem, and efferent fibres transmitting impulses primarily to the muscles. Damage to an individual nerve leads to weakness of the muscles it innervates and sensory loss in the area from which it conveys sensory information. The peripheral nerves occasionally form a dense network or plexus adjacent to the spinal cord (e.g. brachial plexus in the upper limb). The peripheral nerves connect with the spinal cord through foramina between the bones (or **vertebrae**) of the spine (or **vertebral column**), or with the brain through foramina in the skull.

Spinal cord

The **spinal cord** begins at the **foramen magnum**, which is the site in the base of the skull where the lower part of the brainstem (medulla) ends. The spinal cord terminates in the adult at the first lumbar vertebra, and gives rise to 30 pairs (or 31 if the coccygeal nerves are included) of spinal nerves, which exit the spinal cord between the vertebral bones of the spine. The first eight spinal nerves originate from the **cervical spinal cord** with the first pair exiting above the first cervical vertebra and the next 12 spinal nerves originate from the **thoracic or dorsal spinal cord**. The remaining 10 pairs of spinal nerves originate from the lower cord, five from the **lumbar** and five from the **sacral** regions.

The spinal nerves consist of an **anterior or ventral root** that innervates the skeletal muscles, while the **posterior or dorsal root** carries sensation to the spinal cord from the skin that shared a common embryological origin during development with that part of the spinal cord (see Chapter 2). In the case of the dorsal root fibres, they have their cell bodies in the **dorsal root ganglia** which lie just outside the spinal canal.

The spinal cord itself consists of **white matter**, which is that part of it containing the nerve fibres that form the **ascending and descending pathways of the spinal cord**, while the **grey matter** is located in the centre of the spinal cord and contains the cell bodies of the neurones (see Chapter 12).

Brainstem, cranial nerves and cerebellum

The spinal cord gives way to the **brainstem** which lies at the base of the brain and is composed of the **medulla, pons and midbrain** (or mesencephalon as it is sometimes called, although this is strictly a term that should be reserved for this region of the brain in embryonic development) and contains discrete collections of neurones or nuclei for 10 of the 12 cranial nerves (see Chapter 14). The brainstem and the **cerebellum** constitute the structures of the posterior fossa. The cerebellum is connected to the brainstem via three pairs of cerebellar peduncles, and is involved in the coordination of movement (see Chapter 39).

Cerebral hemispheres

The **cerebral hemispheres** are composed of **four major lobes: occipital, parietal, temporal and frontal**. On the medial part of the temporal lobe are a series of structures, including the **hippocampus**, that form the limbic system (see Chapter 46).

The outer layer of the cerebral hemisphere is termed the **cerebral cortex**, and contains neurones that are organized in both horizontal layers and vertical columns (see Chapter 15). The cerebral cortex is interconnected over long distances via pathways that run subcortically. These pathways, together with those that connect the cerebral cortex to the spinal cord, brainstem and nuclei deep within the cerebral hemisphere, constitute **the white matter of the cerebral hemisphere**. These deep nuclei include structures such as the **basal ganglia** (see Chapters 40 and 41) and the **thalamus**.

Meninges

The CNS is enclosed within the skull and vertebral column and separating these structures are a series of membranes known as the **meninges**. The **pia mater** is separated from the delicate **arachnoid membrane** by the subarachnoid space, which in turn is separated from the **dura mater** by the subdural space (see Chapter 18).

Autonomic nervous system

The **ANS** has both a central and peripheral component and is concerned with the innervation of internal and glandular organs (see Chapter 16): it has an important role in the control of the endocrine and homoeostatic systems of the body (see Chapter 17). The peripheral component of the ANS is defined in terms of the **enteric, sympathetic and parasympathetic systems** (see Chapter 16).

The efferent fibres of the ANS originate either from the **intermediate zone** (or **lateral column**) of the spinal cord or specific cranial nerve and sacral nuclei, and synapse in a **ganglion**, the site of which is different for the sympathetic and parasympathetic systems. The afferent fibres from the organs innervated by the ANS pass via the dorsal root to the spinal cord.

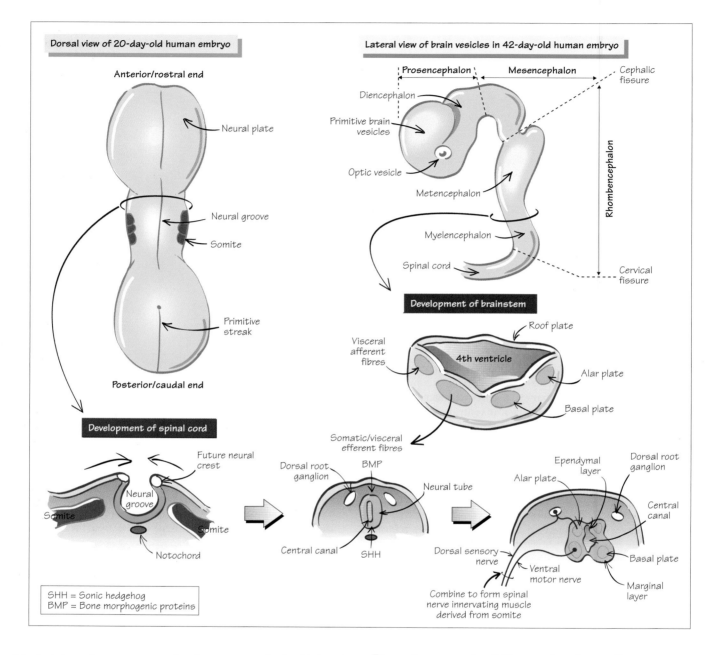

The first signs of nervous system development occur in the third week of gestation, under the influence of secreted factors from the **notochord**, with the formation of a **neural plate** along the dorsal aspect of the embryo. This plate broadens, folds (forming the **neural groove**) and fuses to form the **neural tube** which ultimately gives rise to the brain at its rostral end and the spinal cord caudally. This fusion begins approximately halfway along the neural groove at the level of the fourth somite and continues caudally and rostrally with the closure of the posterior/caudal and anterior/rostral neuropore during the fourth week of gestation. Abnormalities in this process of neuropore closure result in *anencephaly* at the rostral end and certain forms of *spina bifida* at the caudal end (see below).

Development of the spinal cord

The process of neural tube fusion isolates a group of cells termed the **neural crest**. This structure gives rise a range of cells including the **dorsal root ganglia** (DRG) and peripheral components of the ANS. The DRG contain the sensory cell bodies which send their developing axons into the evolving spinal cord and skin. These growing neuronal processes or neurites have an advancing **growth cone** that finds its appropriate target in the periphery and CNS, using a number of cues including cell adhesion molecules and diffusable neurotrophic factors (see Chapter 49).

The neural tube surrounds the neural canal which forms the central canal of the fully developed spinal cord. The tube itself contains the neuroblasts with those adjacent to the canal (**ependymal layer**) dividing and migrating out to the **mantle layer** where they differentiate into neurones and by so doing form the grey matter of the spinal cord (see Chapter 1). The developing processes from the neuroblasts/neurones grow out into the **marginal layer** which therefore ultimately forms the white matter of the spinal cord. The dividing neuroblasts segregate into two discrete populations, the **alar** and **basal plates**, which in turn will form the dorsal and ventral horns of the spinal cord while a small lateral horn of visceral efferent neurones (part of the ANS) develops at their interface in the thoracic and upper lumbar cord (see Chapter 16). This dorsal–ventral patterning relies, at least in part, on secreted factors from the notochord (sonic hedgehog) and dorsally, on bone morphogenic proteins (BMPs).

Development of the brain

The rostral part of the neural tube enlarges before closure with the formation of three **primary brain vesicles (the prosencephalon, mesencephalon and rhombencephalon)** and two **flexures (cervical and cephalic)**. The primary brain vesicles develop into the cerebral hemispheres, brainstem and cerebellum while the neural canal will ultimately form the ventricular system of the brain (see Chapter 18).

The **prosencephalon** consists of the telencephalon which forms the cerebral hemispheres and part of the basal ganglia while the **diencephalon** forms the thalamus, hypothalamus, posterior pituitary and optic nerve and retina.

The neuroblasts again originate adjacent to the neural canal (the ventricular zone) but in this case they migrate not only locally to form the deep subcortical nuclei of the brain, but also out along developing radial glial fibres to form the cerebral cortex (see Chapter 15). This intervening area, which is rich in glial fibres, will ultimately form the white matter of the cerebral hemisphere, with some of the radial glia giving rise to neural precursor cells in the adult brain (see below). The signals involved in the organization of these migrating neurones to and in the cortex are being identified, and defects in these may cause *cortical dysplasia*.

The **mesencephalon** gives rise to the midbrain with the neural canal forming the central aqueduct of Sylvius while the **rhombencephalon** consists of the **metencephalon** which gives rise to the pons and cerebellum and the **myelencephalon** which forms the medulla (see Chapter 13). The brainstem develops in a similar fashion to the spinal cord except the development is in a more mediolateral than anteroposterior direction. Thus, the developing motor nuclei lie medial to the sensory nuclei with a parasympathetic component interposed between the two. This anterolateral expansion therefore explains the organization of the cranial nerve nuclei within the brainstem (see Chapters 13 and 14).

The cerebellum develops from the rhombic lip and adjacent alar layer.

Adult neurogenesis

Until recently it was believed that no new neurones could be born in the adult mammalian brain; however, it is now clear that neural progenitor cells can be found in the adult CNS, including in humans. These cells are predominantly found in the dentate gyrus of the hippocampus (see Chapter 46) and just next to the lateral ventricles in the subventricular zone (SVZ). They may also exist at other sites of the adult CNS but this is contentious. They respond to a number of signals and appear to give rise to functional neurones in the hippocampus and olfactory bulb, with the latter cells migrating from the SVZ to the olfactory bulb via the rostral migratory stream (RMS). They may therefore fulfil a role in certain forms of memory and possibly in mediating the therapeutic effects of some drugs such as antidepressants (see Chapter 54).

Disorders of central nervous system embryogenesis

- *Anencephaly* occurs when there is failure of fusion of the anterior rostral neuropore. The cerebral vesicles fail to develop and thus there is no brain development. The vast majority of fetuses with this abnormality are spontaneously aborted.
- *Spina bifida* refers to any defect at the lower end of the vertebral column and/or spinal cord. The most common form of spina bifida refers to a failure of fusion of the dorsal parts of the lower vertebrae (*spina bifida occulta*). This can be associated with defects in the meninges and neural tissue which may herniate through the defect to form a *meningocoele* and *meningomyelocoele*, respectively. The most serious form of spina bifida is when nervous tissue is directly exposed as a result of a failure in the proper fusion of the posterior/caudal neuropore. Spina bifida is often associated with hydrocephalus (see Chapter 18).

Occasionally, bony defects are found at the base of the skull with the formation of a *meningocoele*. However, unlike the situation at the lower spinal cord, these can often be repaired without any neurological deficit being accrued.
- *Cortical dysplasia* refers to a spectrum of defects that are the result of the abnormal migration of developing cortical neurones. These defects are becoming increasingly recognized with improved imaging of the human CNS, and are now known to be an important cause of *epilepsy* (see Chapter 58).
- Many intrauterine infections (such as rubella), as well as some environmental agents (e.g. radiation), cause major problems in the development of the nervous system. In addition, a large number of rare genetic conditions are associated with defects of CNS development but these lie beyond the scope of this book.

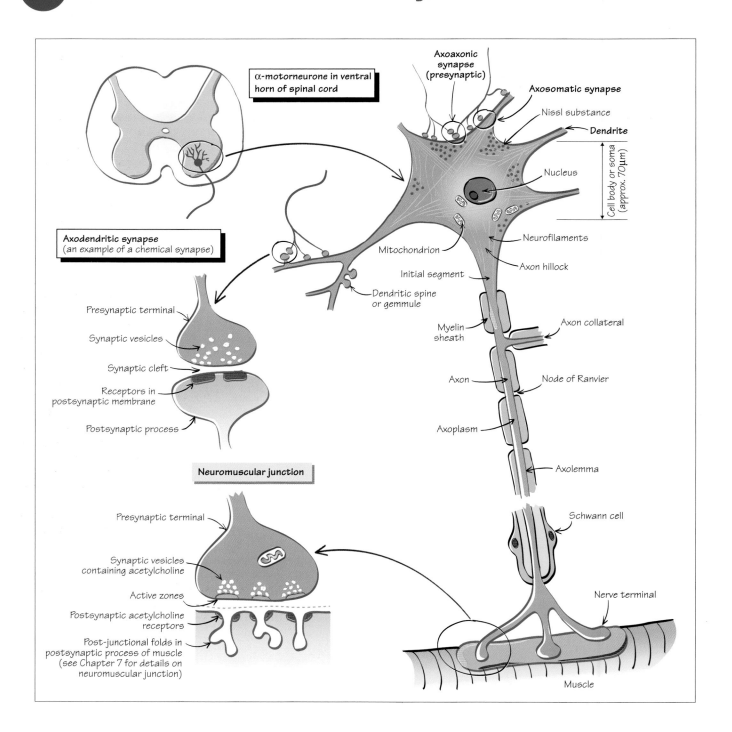

There are two major classes of cells in the nervous system: the neuro-glial cells and neurones, with the latter making up only 10–20% of the whole population. The neurones are specialized for excitation and nerve impulse conduction (see Chapters 5, 6 and 8), and communicate with each other by means of the synapse (see Chapter 7) and so act as the structural and functional unit of the nervous system.

Neurones

The **cell body (soma)** is that part of the neurone containing the nucleus and surrounding cytoplasm. It is the focus of cellular metabolism, and houses most of the neurone's intracellular organelles (**mitochondria**, Golgi apparatus and peroxisomes). It is associated typically with two types of neuronal process: the **dendrites** and **axon**. Most neurones also contain the granular basophilic staining, **Nissl substance**, which is composed of granular endoplasmic reticulum and ribosomes and is responsible for protein synthesis. This is located within the cell body and dendritic processes but is absent from the **axon hillock** and axon itself, for reasons that are not clear. In addition, throughout the cell body and processes are **neurofilaments** which are important in maintaining the architecture or cytoskeleton of the neurone. Furthermore, two other fibrillary structures within the neurone are important in this respect: microtubules and microfilaments, structures that are also important for axoplasmic flow (see below) and axonal growth.

The **dendrites** are neuronal cell processes that taper from the soma outwards, branch profusely and are responsible for conveying information towards the soma from **synapses** on the dendritic tree (**axodendritic synapses**; see also Chapter 8). Most neurones have many dendrites (**multipolar neurones**) and while some inputs synapse directly on the dendrite, some do so via small **dendritic spines or gemmules**. Thus, the primary role of dendrites is to increase the surface area for synapse formation allowing integration of a large number of inputs that are relayed to the cell body. In contrast, the **axon**, of which there is only one per neurone, conducts information away from the soma towards the **nerve terminal** and synapses (see Chapter 8). Although there is only one axon per neurone, it can branch to give several processes. This branching occurs close to the soma in the case of sensory neurones (**pseudo-unipolar** neurones; see Chapter 22), but more typically occurs close to the synaptic target of the axon. The axon originates from the soma at the **axon hillock** where the **initial segment** of the axon emerges. This is the most excitable part of a neurone because of its high density of sodium channels, and so is the site of initiation of the action potential (see Chapter 6).

All neurones are bounded by a lipid bilayer (**cell membrane**) within which proteins are located, some of which form ion channels (see Chapter 5); others form receptors to specific chemicals that are released by neurones (see Chapters 7 and 9) and others act as ion pumps moving ions across the membrane against their electrochemical gradient, e.g. Na^+–K^+ exchange pump (see Chapter 6). The axonal surface membrane is known as the **axolemma** and the cytoplasm contained within it, the **axoplasm**. The ion channels within the axolemma imbue the axon with its ability to conduct action potentials while the axoplasm contains neurofilaments, microtubules and mitochondria. These latter organelles are not only responsible for maintaining the ionic gradients necessary for action potential production, but also allow for the transport and recycling of proteins away from (and to a lesser extent towards) the soma to the nerve terminal. This **axoplasmic flow or axonal transport** is either slow (~1 mm/day) or fast (~100–400 mm/day) and is not

only important in permitting normal neuronal/synaptic activity but may also be important for neuronal survival and development and as such may be abnormal in some neurodegenerative disorders such as motorneurone disease as well as disorders associated with abnormalities in the protein τ (see Chapter 57).

Many axons are surrounded by a layer of lipid, or **myelin sheath**, which acts as an electrical insulator. This myelin sheath alters the conducting properties of the axon, and allows for rapid action potential propagation without a loss of signal integrity (see Chapter 8). This is achieved by means of gaps, or **nodes (of Ranvier)**, in the myelin sheath where the axolemma contains many ion channels (typically Na^+ channels) which are directly exposed to the tissue fluid. The nodes of Ranvier are also those sites from which axonal branches originate, and these branches are termed **axon collaterals**. The myelin sheath encompasses the axon just beyond the initial segment and finishes just prior to its terminal arborization. The myelin sheath is formed by **Schwann cells** in the peripheral nervous system (PNS) and by **oligodendrocytes** in the central nervous system (CNS) (see Chapter 4), with many CNS axons being ensheathed by a single oligodendrocyte while in the PNS one Schwann cell provides myelin for one internode.

The **synapse** is the junction where a neurone meets another cell, which in the case of the CNS is another neurone. In the PNS the target can be muscle, glandular cells or other organs. The typical synapse in the nervous system is a **chemical** one, which is composed of a **presynaptic nerve terminal (bouton or end-bulb)**, and a **synaptic cleft** which physically separates the nerve terminal from the **postsynaptic membrane** and across which the chemical or neurotransmitter from the presynaptic terminal must diffuse (see Chapter 7). This synapse is typically between an axon of one neurone and the dendrite of another (**axodendritic synapse**) although synapses are found where the point of contact between the axon and the postsynaptic cell is either at the level of the cell body (**axosomatic synapses**) or, less frequently, the presynaptic nerve terminal (**axoaxonic synapse**; see Chapter 8). A few synapses within the CNS do not possess these features but are low-resistance junctions (gap junctions) and are termed **electrical synapses**. These synapses allow for rapid conduction of action potentials without any integration and as such tend to enable populations of cells to fire together or in synchrony (see Chapters 7 and 58). They may also be important in the coupling of activity across cortical areas which may be important in some of the synchronized responses seen in the brain in sleep-wakefulness (see Chapter 44 and 45).

The specific loss of neurones is seen in a number of neurological disorders, and those diseases in which this is the primary event are discussed in Chapter 57.

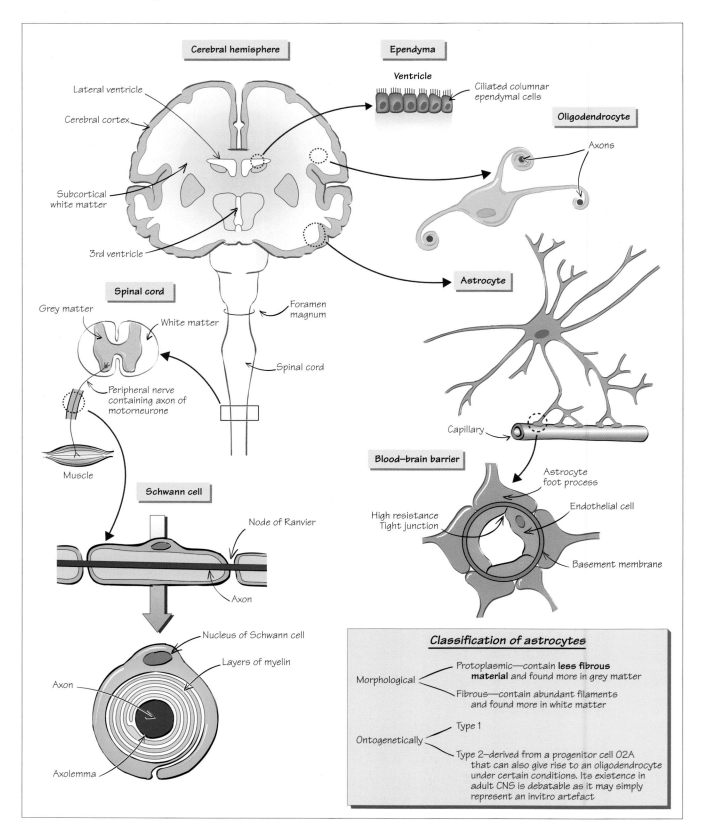

Cerebral hemisphere

Ependyma

Ventricle

Lateral ventricle

Cerebral cortex

Ciliated columnar ependymal cells

Oligodendrocyte

Axons

Subcortical white matter

3rd ventricle

Astrocyte

Spinal cord

Grey matter

White matter

Foramen magnum

Spinal cord

Peripheral nerve containing axon of motorneurone

Muscle

Capillary

Blood–brain barrier

Astrocyte foot process

Endothelial cell

High resistance Tight junction

Basement membrane

Schwann cell

Node of Ranvier

Axon

Nucleus of Schwann cell

Layers of myelin

Axon

Axolemma

Classification of astrocytes

Morphological — Protoplasmic—contain **less fibrous material** and found more in grey matter

— Fibrous—contain abundant filaments and found more in white matter

Ontogenetically — Type 1

— Type 2–derived from a progenitor cell O2A that can also give rise to an oligodendrocyte under certain conditions. Its existence in adult CNS is debatable as it may simply represent an invitro artefact

There are four main classes of neuroglial cells within the central nervous system (CNS): astrocytes, oligodendrocytes, ependymal cells and microglia, all of which subserve different functions. In contrast, in the peripheral nervous system (PNS), Schwann cells are the only example of neuroglia and are involved in myelination and facilitating axonal regeneration.

Astrocytes are small stellate cells that are found throughout the CNS and classified either morphologically or ontogenetically (see figure). They subserve many important functions within the CNS and are not simply passive support elements.
• They form a structural and supporting framework for neuronal cells and capillaries by virtue of their cytoplasmic processes, which end in close apposition not only to neurones but also to capillaries. In this respect they form the glia limitans—where the astrocytic foot processes cover the basal laminae around blood vessels and at the pia mater.
• They maintain the integrity of the **blood–brain barrier (BBB)**, by promoting the formation of high-resistance junctions between brain capillary endothelial cells (see Chapter 18).
• They are capable of taking up, storing and releasing some neurotransmitters (e.g. glutamate, γ-aminobutyric acid [GABA]) and thus may be an important adjunct in chemical neurotransmission within the CNS.
• They can take up and disperse excessive ion concentration in the extracellular fluid, especially K^+.
• They participate in neuronal guidance during development (see Chapter 15), and may also be important in the response to injury (see Chapter 50) and in directing the fate of neural precursor cells in the adult hippocampus to neurones.
• They may have a role in presenting antigen to the immune system in situations where the CNS and BBB are damaged (see Chapter 59).

The most common clinical disorder of astrocytes is their abnormal proliferation in tumours called *astrocytomas*. These tumours produce effects by compressing adjacent CNS tissue and this presents as an evolving neurological deficit (with or without epileptic seizures) depending on its site of origin within the CNS. In adults, the tumours most commonly arise in the white matter of the cerebral hemispheres.

Oligodendrocytes are responsible for the myelination of CNS neurones, and are therefore found in large numbers in the white matter. Each oligodendrocyte forms internodal myelin for 3–50 fibres and also surrounds many other fibres without forming myelin sheaths. In addition, they have a number of molecules associated with them that are inhibitory to axonal growth, and thus contribute to the failure of damaged adult CNS neurones and their axons to regenerate (see Chapter 50).

Clinical disorders of oligodendrocyte function cause central demyelination which is seen in a number of conditions including *multiple sclerosis* (see Chapter 59), while abnormal proliferation of oligodendrocytes produces a slow-growing tumour (an *oligodendroglioma*) which tends to present with epileptic seizures (see Chapter 58).

Ependymal cells are important in facilitating the movement of cerebrospinal fluid (CSF) as well as interacting with astrocytes to form a barrier separating the ventricles and the CSF from the neuronal environment. They also line the central canal in the spinal cord (see Chapter 12). These ependymal cells are termed ependymocytes to distinguish them from those ependymal cells that are involved in the formation of CSF (the choroid plexus) and those that transport substances from the CSF to blood (tanycytes). Tumours of the ependyma (*ependymomas or choroid plexus papillomas*) occur either in the ventricles where they tend to produce *hydrocephalus* (see Chapter 18) or spinal cord where they cause local destruction of the neural structures.

Microglial cells (not shown on figure) are the tissue macrophages of the brain, and are found throughout the white and grey matter of the CNS. They are phagocytic in nature and are important in mediating immune responses within the CNS (see Chapter 59). There is also recent interest in their role in mediating an inflammatory component to the neurodegenerative processes seen in some disorders of the CNS, such as Parkinson's disease (see Chapter 41 and 57).

Schwann cells are found only in the PNS and are responsible for the myelination of peripheral nerves by a process that involves the wrapping of the cell around the axon. Thus, the final myelin sheath is composed of multiple layers of Schwann cell membrane in which the cytoplasm has been extruded. Unlike oligodendrocytes, one Schwann cell envelops one axon and provides myelin for one internode. In addition, Schwann cells are important in the regeneration of damaged peripheral axons, in contrast to the largely inhibitory functions of the central neuroglial cells (see Chapters 49 and 50). A number of genetic and inflammatory neuropathies are associated with the loss of peripheral myelin (as opposed to the loss of axons), which results in peripheral nerve dysfunction (*demyelinating neuropathies*; see Chapters 6 and 60). In addition, benign tumours of Schwann cells can occur (*schwannomas*), especially in certain genetic conditions such as *neurofibromatosis type I*, where there is the loss of the tumour suppressor gene, neurofibromin. These tumours are typically asymptomatic but if they arise in areas of limited space they can produce symptoms by compression of the neighbouring neural structures; e.g. at the cerebellopontine angle in the brainstem or spinal root (see Chapters 12–14 and 39). Finally, there are a group of rare disorders, typically inherited, that cause a central abnormality of myelination, which together are called leucodystophies.

5 Ion channels

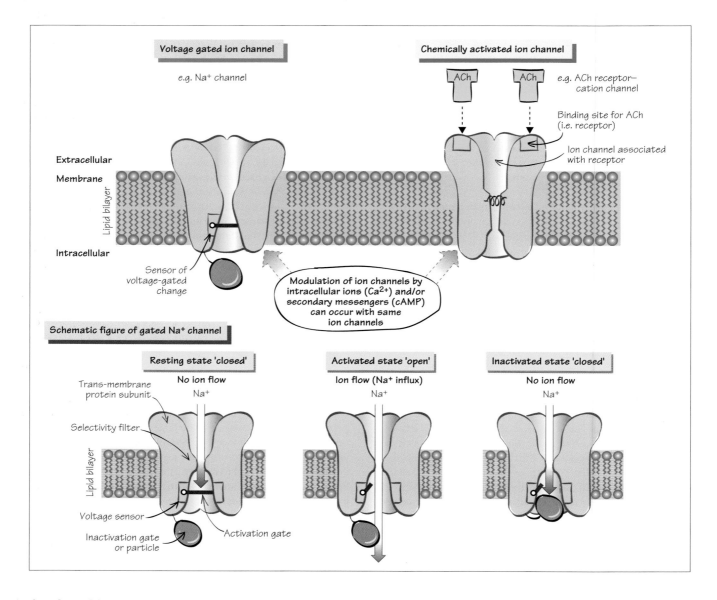

An **ion channel** is a protein macromolecule that spans a biological membrane and allows ions to pass from one side of the membrane to the other. The ions move in a direction determined by the electrochemical gradient across the membrane. In general, ions will tend to flow from an area of high concentration to one of low concentration, but in the presence of a voltage gradient it is possible for there to be no ion flow even with unequal concentrations. The ion channel itself can be open or closed. Opening can be achieved either by changing the voltage across the membrane (e.g. a depolarization or the arrival of an action potential) or by the binding of a chemical substance to a receptor in or near the channel. The two types of channel are called **voltage gated** (or **voltage sensitive**) and **chemically activated** (or **ligand gated**) channels, respectively. However, this distinction is somewhat artificial as a number of voltage sensitive channels can be modulated by neurotransmitters as well as by Ca^{2+}. Furthermore, some ion channels are not opened by voltage changes or chemical messengers but are directly opened by mechanical stretch or pressure (e.g. the somatosensory and auditory receptors; see Chapters 21, 22, 28 and 30).

The most important property of ion channels is that they imbue the neurone with electrical excitability (see Chapter 6) and while they are found in all parts of the neurone, and to a lesser extent in neuroglial cells, they are also seen in a host of non-neural cells.

All biological membranes, including the neuronal membrane, are composed of a lipid bilayer that has a high electrical resistance, i.e. ions will not readily flow through it. Therefore, in order for ions to move across a membrane, it is necessary to have either 'pores' (ion channels) in the lipid bilayer or 'carriers' that will collect the ions from one side of the membrane and carry them across to the other side where they are released. In neurones, the rate of ion transfer necessary for signal transmission is too fast for any carrier system and so ion channels (or 'pores') are employed by neurones for the transfer of ions across the membrane.

The fundamental properties of an ion channel are as follows:
- It is composed of a number of protein subunits that traverse the membrane and allow ions to cross from one side to the other—a **transmembrane pore**.
- The channel so formed must be able to move from a **closed** to an **open** state and back, although intermediate steps may be required.
- It must be able to open in response to specific stimuli. Most channels possess a sensor of voltage change and so open in response to a depolarizing voltage, i.e. one that moves the resting membrane potential from its resting value of approximately -70 to -80 mV to a less negative value.

In contrast, some channels, especially those found at synapses, are not opened by a voltage change but by a chemical, e.g. acetylcholine (ACh). These channels have a **receptor** for that chemical and the binding of the chemical to this receptor leads to channel opening. However, many channels possess both voltage and chemical sensors and the presence of an intracellular ion or secondary messenger molecule (e.g. cyclic adenosine monophosphate [cAMP]) leads to a **modulation** of the ion flow across the membrane that the voltage-dependent process has produced.

Activation of the voltage sensor or chemical receptor leads to the opening of a '**gate**' within the channel which allows ions to flow through the channel. The channel is then closed by either a process of **deactivation** (which is simply the reversal of the opening of the gate) or **inactivation** which involves a **second gate** moving into the channel more slowly than the activation gate moves out, so that there is a time when there is no gate in the channel and ions can flow through it.

The flow of ions through the channel can be either **selective or non-selective**. If the channel is selective then it only allows certain ions through and it achieves this by means of a '**filter**'. The selectivity filter is based on energetic considerations (thermodynamically) and gives the channel its name, e.g. sodium channel. However, certain channels are non-selective in that they allow many different types of similarly charged ions through, e.g. ACh cation channel.

The overall description of an ion channel is in terms of a number of different physical measures. The net flow of ions through a channel is termed the **current**; while the **conductance** is defined as the reciprocal of resistance (current/voltage) and represents the ease with which the ions can pass through the membrane. **Permeability**, on the other hand, is defined as the rate of transport of a substance or ion through the membrane for a given concentration difference.

There are many different types of ion channels and even within a single family of ion-specific channels there are multiple subtypes, e.g. there are at least five different types of potassium channels.

The number and type of ion channels governs the response characteristics of the cell. In the case of neurones, this is expressed in terms of the rate of action potential generation and its response to synaptic inputs (see Chapters 6–8, 46 and 58).

Clinical disorders of ion channels

A number of pharmacological agents work at the level of ion channels, including local anaesthetics and some antiepileptic drugs. However, in recent years a number of neurological disorders, primarily involving muscle, have been found to be caused by mutations in the sodium and chloride ion channels. These conditions include various forms of *myotonia* (delayed relaxation of skeletal muscle following voluntary contraction, i.e. an inability to let go of objects easily) and various forms of *periodic paralyses* in which patients develop a transient flaccid weakness which can be either partial or generalized. Furthermore, certain forms of familial hemiplegic *migraine* and cerebellar dysfunction (see Chapter 39) are associated with abnormalities in the Ca^{2+} channel, and some forms of *epilepsy* (see Chapter 58) may be caused by a disorder of specific ion channels. In other disorders there is a redistribution or exposing of normally non-functioning ion channels. This commonly occurs next to the node of Ranvier as a result of central demyelination in *multiple sclerosis* and peripheral demyelination in the *Guillain–Barré syndrome*, and results in an impairment in action potential propagation (see Chapters 6 and 59). Finally, in some conditions, antibodies are produced in the body (sometimes in response to a tumour) which react with voltage gated ion channels giving disorders in the CNS (e.g. limbic encephalitis and anti-voltage gated potassium channels) as well as in the PNS (Lambert–Eaton myasthenic syndrome and anti-voltage gated calcium channels).

6 The resting membrane and action potential

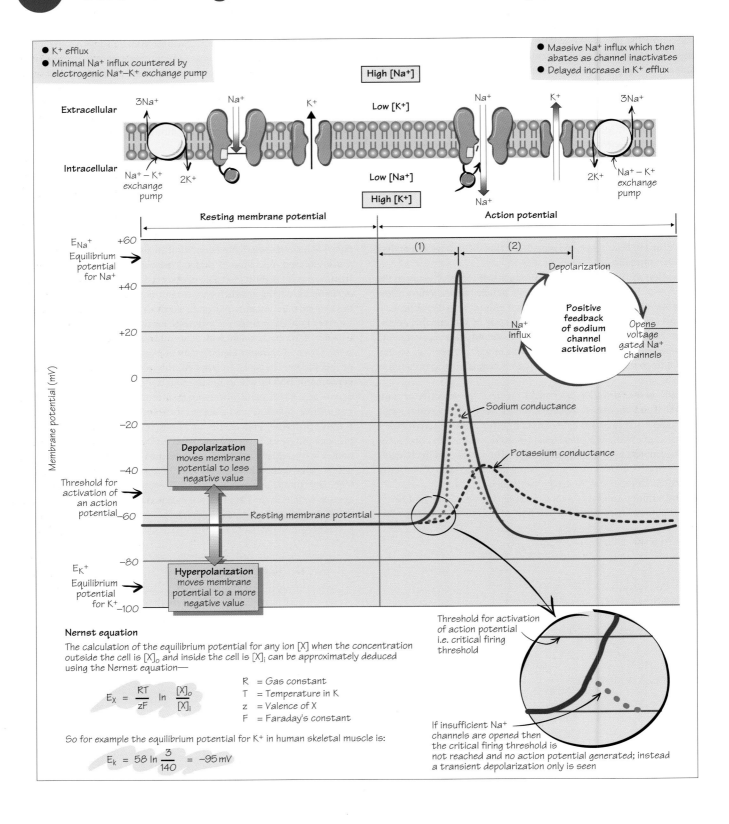

- K$^+$ efflux
- Minimal Na$^+$ influx countered by electrogenic Na$^+$–K$^+$ exchange pump

- Massive Na$^+$ influx which then abates as channel inactivates
- Delayed increase in K$^+$ efflux

High [Na$^+$]

Low [K$^+$]

Low [Na$^+$]

High [K$^+$]

Extracellular

Intracellular

3Na$^+$ Na$^+$ K$^+$ Na$^+$ K$^+$ 3Na$^+$

Na$^+$ – K$^+$ exchange pump   2K$^+$ 2K$^+$ Na$^+$ – K$^+$ exchange pump   Na$^+$

Resting membrane potential

Action potential

(1)   (2)

Depolarization

Positive feedback of sodium channel activation

Na$^+$ influx   Opens voltage gated Na$^+$ channels

E_{Na^+} Equilibrium potential for Na$^+$ +60

+40

+20

0

−20

−40

Threshold for activation of an action potential   −60

−80

E_{K^+} Equilibrium potential for K$^+$ −100

Membrane potential (mV)

Depolarization moves membrane potential to less negative value

Hyperpolarization moves membrane potential to a more negative value

Resting membrane potential

Sodium conductance

Potassium conductance

Threshold for activation of action potential i.e. critical firing threshold

If insufficient Na$^+$ channels are opened then the critical firing threshold is not reached and no action potential generated; instead a transient depolarization only is seen

Nernst equation

The calculation of the equilibrium potential for any ion [X] when the concentration outside the cell is [X]$_o$ and inside the cell is [X]$_i$ can be approximately deduced using the Nernst equation—

$$E_X = \frac{RT}{zF} \ln \frac{[X]_o}{[X]_i}$$

R = Gas constant
T = Temperature in K
z = Valence of X
F = Faraday's constant

So for example the equilibrium potential for K$^+$ in human skeletal muscle is:

$$E_k = 58 \ln \frac{3}{140} = -95\,mV$$

Resting membrane potential

In the resting state, the neuronal cell membrane is relatively impermeable to ions. This is important in the generation of the **resting membrane potential**. The major intracellular ion is potassium, compared to sodium in the extracellular fluid, and so the natural flow of ions according to their concentration gradients is for K^+ to leave the cell (or efflux) and for Na^+ to enter (or influx). The movement of positive ions out of the cell leads to the generation of a negative membrane potential or **hyperpolarization**, while the converse is true for positive ion influx (a process of **depolarization**). However, the resting membrane is relatively impermeable to Na^+ ions while being relatively permeable to K^+ ions. At rest therefore, K^+ will tend to efflux from the cell down its concentration gradient, leaving excess negative charge behind, and this will continue until the chemical concentration gradient driving K^+ out of the cell is exactly offset by the electrical potential difference generated by this efflux (the membrane potential) drawing K^+ back into the cell. The membrane potential at which this steady state is achieved is the **equilibrium potential** for K^+ (E_{K^+}) and can be derived using the **Nernst equation** (see figure for details). In fact, the measured resting membrane potential in axons is slightly more positive than expected because there is some small permeability to Na^+ of the membrane in the resting state. The small Na^+ influx is countered by an adenosine triphosphate (ATP) dependent **Na^+–K^+ exchange pump** which is itself slightly electrogenic. This pump is essential in maintaining the ionic gradients, and is electrogenic by virtue of the fact that it pumps out three Na^+ ions for every two K^+ ions brought in. It makes only a small contribution to the level of the resting membrane potential.

Action potential generation

One of the fundamental features of the nervous system is its ability to generate and conduct electrical impulses (see Chapters 8 and 21). These can take the form of generator potentials, synaptic potentials and action potentials—the latter being defined as a single electrical impulse passing down an axon. This **action potential (nerve impulse or spike)** is an **all-or-nothing phenomenon**, that is to say once the threshold stimulus intensity is reached an action potential will be generated. Therefore information in the nervous system is coded by frequency of firing rather than size of the action potential (see Chapter 20). The threshold stimulus intensity is defined as that value at which the net inward current (which is largely determined by Na^+ ions) is just greater than the net outward current (which is largely carried by K^+ ions), and is typically around $-55\,mV$ (**critical firing threshold**). This occurs most readily in the region of the axon hillock where there is the highest density of Na^+ channels, and is thus the site of action potential initiation in the neurone. However, if the threshold is not reached the graded depolarization will not generate an action potential and the signal will not be propagated along the axon.

The sequence of events in the generation of an action potential are as follows:

1 The depolarizing voltage activates the voltage sensitive Na^+ channels in the neuronal membrane which allows some Na^+ ions to flow down their electrochemical gradient (increased Na^+ conductance). This depolarizes the membrane still further, opening more Na^+ channels in a **positive feedback loop**. When sufficient Na^+ channels are opened to produce an inward current greater than that generated by the K^+ efflux, there is rapid opening of all the Na^+ channels producing a large influx of Na^+ which depolarizes the membrane towards the **equilibrium potential for Na^+** (approximately $+55\,mV$). The spike of the action potential is therefore generated, but fails to reach the equilibrium potential for Na^+ because of the persistent and increasing K^+ efflux.

2 The falling phase of the action potential then follows as the voltage sensitive Na^+ channels become inactivated (see Chapter 5). This inactivation is voltage dependent, in that it is in response to the depolarizing stimulus, but has slower kinetics than the activation process and so occurs later (see Chapter 5). During this falling phase, a voltage dependent K^+ current becomes important as its activation by the depolarization of the membrane has even slower kinetics than sodium channel inactivation. This voltage activated K^+ channel leads to a brief period of membrane hyperpolarization before it deactivates and the membrane potential is returned to the resting state.

Immediately after the spike of the action potential there is a **refractory period** when the neurone is either inexcitable (**absolute refractory period**) or only activated to submaximal responses by suprathreshold stimuli (**relative refractory period**). The absolute refractory period occurs at the time of maximal Na^+ channel inactivation, while the relative refractory period occurs at a later time when most of the Na^+ channels have returned to their resting state but the voltage activated K^+ current is well developed. The refractory period has two important implications for action potential generation and conduction. First, action potentials can be conducted only in one direction, away from the site of its generation and, secondly, they can be generated only up to certain limiting frequencies (see Chapter 20).

The original description of the mechanism of generation of the action potential was by Hodgkin and Huxley in the squid giant axon in the 1950s but subsequently it has been confirmed in many other cells and neurones. This, together with the discovery of a large number of ion channels, has meant that many modifications relating to the generation and characteristics of action potentials in neurones and other cells have been described.

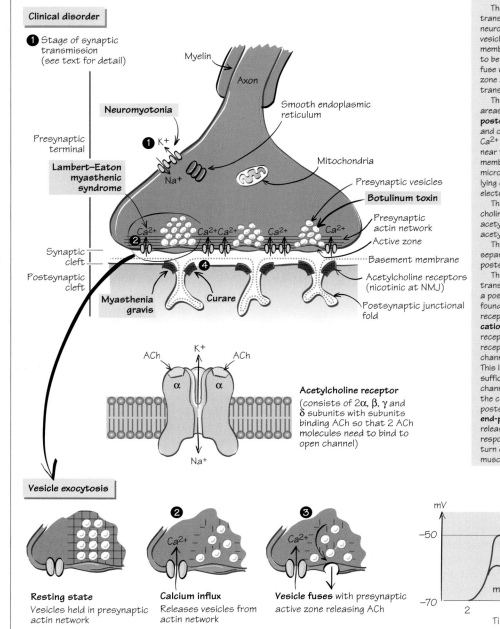

The **presynaptic vesicles** contain the neuro-transmitter, which is acetylcholine (ACh) at the neuromuscular junction (NMJ). In addition the vesicles contain ATP and a number of specific membrane-associated proteins which allow them to be drawn to the presynaptic active zone, to fuse with the presynaptic membrane at the active zone and to be recycled and loaded with new transmitter.

The **presynaptic active zones** are specialized areas for vesicle release that lie opposite the **postsynaptic secondary (or junctional) folds**, and contain a high density of voltage-dependent Ca^{2+} channels. Mitochondria and vesicles cluster near these darkly stained patches in the terminal membrane which are characterized on electron microscopy by a double row of synaptic vesicles lying close to the membrane on both sides of an electron-dense structure.

The **cleft substance** is found only at the cholinergic NMJ, and contains the enzyme acetylcholinesterase (AChE) which inactivates acetylcholine by hydrolysis.

The **synaptic cleft** is around 50 nm wide and separates the presynaptic terminal from the postsynaptic membrane.

The **acetylcholine receptors (AChRs)** that translate the released neurotransmitter into a postsynaptic electrical event are preferentially found between the junctional folds. These receptors are associated with a **non-selective cation** channel. The binding of ACh to this receptor induces a conformational change in the receptor leading to the opening of this channel, with an influx of Na^+ and an efflux of K^+. This leads to membrane depolarization which, if sufficient, activates voltage-dependent ion channels. In the case of the NMJ, the release of the contents of a single vesicle produces a small postsynaptic depolarization, called a **miniature end-plate potential (mepp)**. If more vesicles are released the mepps summate to give a larger response or **end-plate potential (epp)** which in turn can generate an action potential in the muscle.

Acetylcholine receptor (consists of 2α, β, γ and δ subunits with subunits binding ACh so that 2 ACh molecules need to bind to open channel)

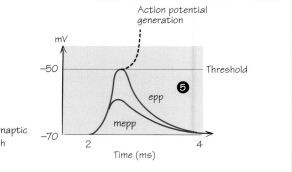

Resting state
Vesicles held in presynaptic actin network

Calcium influx
Releases vesicles from actin network

Vesicle fuses with presynaptic active zone releasing ACh

Sherrington in 1897 coined the term **'synapse'** to mean the junction of two neurones. Much of the work on the synapse has been carried out with the cholinergic **neuromuscular junction (NMJ)**, although it appears that this chemical synapse is similar in its mode of action to those found in the central nervous system (CNS). The chemical synapse is the predominant synapse type found in the nervous system, but electrical synapses are found in certain sites, e.g. glial cells (see Chapter 4).

Neuromuscular transmission (a model for synaptic transmission)

The sequence of events at a chemical synapse is as follows:

• The arrival of the action potential leads to the depolarization of the presynaptic terminal (labelled (**1**) on figure) with the opening of **voltage-dependent Ca^{2+} channels** in the **active zones** of the presynaptic terminal and subsequent Ca^{2+} influx (**2**) (this is the stage that represents the major delay in synaptic transmission).

- The influx of Ca^{2+} leads to the phosphorylation and alteration of a number of presynaptic calcium-binding proteins (some of which are found in the vesicle membrane) which liberates the **vesicle** from its **presynaptic actin network** allowing it to bind to the **presynaptic membrane (3)**. These proteins include various different soluble NSF attachment proteins (SNAPs) and SNAP receptors (SNAREs).
- The fusion of the two hemichannels (presynaptic vesicle and presynaptic membrane) leads to the formation of a small pore that rapidly expands with the release of vesicular contents into the **synaptic cleft**. The vesicle membrane can then be recycled by **endocytosis** into the presynaptic terminal, either by a non-selective or more selective clathrin-mediated process.
- Most of the released neurotransmitter then diffuses across the synaptic cleft and binds to the **postsynaptic receptor (4)**. Some transmitter molecules diffuse out of the synaptic cleft and are lost, while others are inactivated before they have time to bind to the postsynaptic membrane receptor. This **inactivation** is essential for the synapse to function normally and, although enzymatic degradation of acetylcholine (ACh) is employed at the NMJ, other synapses employ uptake mechanisms with the recycling of the transmitter into the presynaptic neurone (see Chapter 9).
- The activation of the postsynaptic receptor leads to a change in the postsynaptic membrane potential. Each vesicle contains a certain amount or quantum of neurotransmitter, whose release generates a small postsynaptic potential change of a fixed size—the **miniature end-plate potential (mepp)**. The release of transmitter from several vesicles leads to mepp summation and the generation of a larger depolarization or **end-plate potential (epp)** which, if sufficiently large, will reach threshold for action potential generation in the postsynaptic muscle fibre **(5)**.

This **vesicle hypothesis** has been criticized, because not all CNS synapses contain their neurotransmitters in vesicles and because electrical synapses are found in some neural networks. Alternative theories have therefore been put forward that invoke either molecules to carry the neurotransmitter across the presynaptic membrane or pores that open in the presynaptic membrane in response to a calcium influx. There is little evidence in favour of either of these theories.

Disorders of neuromuscular transmission

There are a number of naturally occurring toxins that can affect the NMJ.
- **Curare** binds to the acetylcholine receptor (AChR) and prevents ACh from acting on it and so induces paralysis. This is exploited clinically in the use of curare derivatives for muscle paralysis in certain forms of surgery.
- **Botulinum toxin** prevents the release of ACh presynaptically. In this case an exotoxin from the bacterium *Clostridium botulinum* binds to the presynaptic membrane of the ACh synapse and prevents the quantal release of ACh. The accidental ingestion of this toxin in cases of food poisoning produces paralysis and autonomic failure (see Chapter 16). However, the toxin can be used therapeutically in small quantities by injecting it into muscles that are abnormally overactive in certain forms of focal *dystonia*—a condition in which a part of the body is held in a fixed abnormal posture by overactive muscular activity (see Chapter 41). It is also used in cosmetic surgery to get rid of wrinkles.

A number of neurological conditions affect the NMJ selectively. These include *myasthenia gravis*, *the Lambert–Eaton myasthenic syndrome (LEMS)* and *neuromyotonia or Isaac's syndrome*. In *neuromyotonia* the patient complains of muscle cramps and stiffness as a result of continuous motor activity in the muscle. This is often caused by an antibody directed against the presynaptic voltage gated K^+ channel, so the nerve terminal is always in a state of depolarization with transmitter release. In contrast, in **LEMS** there is an antibody directed against the presynaptic Ca^{2+} channel, so that on repeated activation of the synapse there is a steady increase in Ca^{2+} influx as the blocking antibody is competitively overcome by exogenous Ca^{2+}. The patient complains of weakness, especially of the proximal muscles, which transiently improves on exercise. *Myasthenia gravis*, on the other hand, is caused by an antibody against the AChR, and patients complain of weakness that increases with exercise (fatiguability) involving the eyes, throat and limbs. This weakness is because the number of AChR are reduced and the presynaptic release of ACh competes for the few available receptors. More recently, a second antibody has been recognized in myasthenia gravis in patients without antibodies to the AChR. This antibody is directed to a muscle specific kinase (MUSK), although exactly how this causes the syndrome is not fully known.

Electrical synapses

Electrical transmission occurs at a small number of sites in the brain. The presence of fast conducting gap junctions promotes the rapid and widespread propagation of electrical activity and thus may be important in synchronizing some aspects of cortical function (see Chapter 15). The abnormal absence of gap junctions in Schwann cells leads to one form of peripheral hereditary motor sensory neuropathy (HMSN).

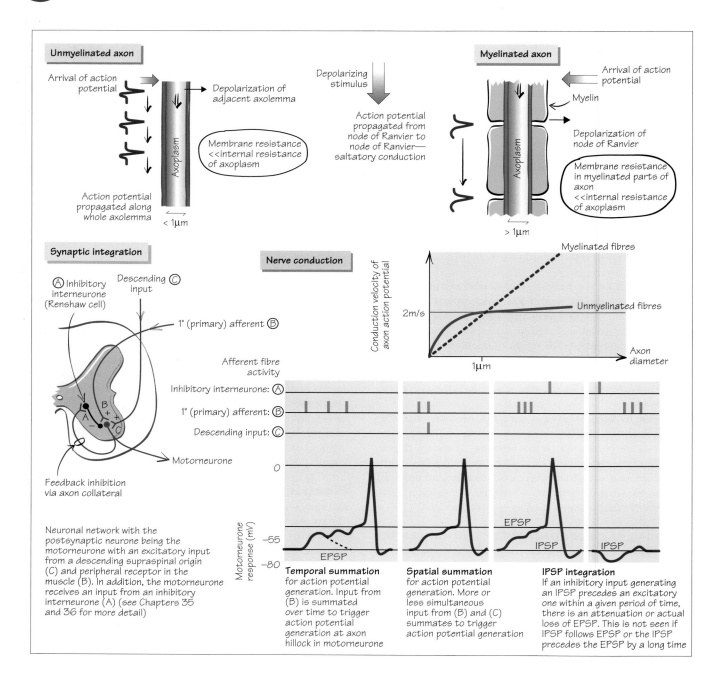

Unmyelinated axon

Arrival of action potential

→ Depolarization of adjacent axolemma

Axoplasm

Membrane resistance <<internal resistance of axoplasm

Action potential propagated along whole axolemma

< 1µm

Depolarizing stimulus

Action potential propagated from node of Ranvier to node of Ranvier— saltatory conduction

Myelinated axon

Arrival of action potential

Myelin

Axoplasm

Depolarization of node of Ranvier

Membrane resistance in myelinated parts of axon <<internal resistance of axoplasm

> 1µm

Synaptic integration

(A) Inhibitory interneurone (Renshaw cell)

Descending (C) input

1° (primary) afferent (B)

Motorneurone

Feedback inhibition via axon collateral

Neuronal network with the postsynaptic neurone being the motorneurone with an excitatory input from a descending supraspinal origin (C) and peripheral receptor in the muscle (B). In addition, the motorneurone receives an input from an inhibitory interneurone (A) (see Chapters 35 and 36 for more detail)

Nerve conduction

Conduction velocity of axon action potential

Myelinated fibres

2m/s

Unmyelinated fibres

Axon diameter

1µm

Afferent fibre activity

Inhibitory interneurone: (A)

1° (primary) afferent: (B)

Descending input: (C)

0

Motorneurone response (mV)

−55

−80

EPSP

EPSP

EPSP

IPSP

IPSP

Temporal summation for action potential generation. Input from (B) is summated over time to trigger action potential generation at axon hillock in motorneurone

Spatial summation for action potential generation. More or less simultaneous input from (B) and (C) summates to trigger action potential generation

IPSP integration If an inhibitory input generating an IPSP precedes an excitatory one within a given period of time, there is an attenuation or actual loss of EPSP. This is not seen if IPSP follows EPSP or the IPSP precedes the EPSP by a long time

Nerve conduction

Action potential propagation is achieved by local current spread and is made possible by the large safety factor in the generation of an action potential as a consequence of the positive feedback of Na+ channel activation in the rising phase of the nerve impulse (see Chapter 6). However, the use of local current spread does set constraints, not only on the velocity of nerve conduction; it also influences the fidelity of the signal being conducted. The nervous system overcomes these difficulties by insulating nerve fibres above a given diameter with myelin which is periodically interrupted by the nodes of Ranvier.

In **unmyelinated axons** an action potential at one site leads to depolarization of the membrane immediately in front and theoretically behind it, although the membrane at this site is in its refractory state and so the action potential is only conducted in one direction (see Chapter 6). The current preferentially passes across the membrane (because of the high internal resistance of the axoplasm) and is greatest at the site closest to the action potential.

However, while nerve impulse conduction is feasible and accurate in unmyelinated axons, especially in the very small-diameter fibres where the internal axoplasmic resistance is very high, it is nevertheless slow.

Conduction velocity can therefore be increased by either increasing the axon diameter (of which the best example is the squid giant axon with a diameter of ~1 mm) or insulating the axon using a high-resistance substance such as the lipid-rich myelin.

Conduction in **myelinated fibres** follows exactly the same sequence of events as in unmyelinated fibres, but with a crucial difference: the advancing action potential encounters a high-resistance low-capacitance structure in the form of a nerve fibre wrapped in myelin. The depolarizing current therefore passes along the axoplasm until it reaches a low-resistance **node of Ranvier** with its high density of Na^+ channels and an action potential is generated at this site. The action potential therefore appears to be conducted down the fibre, from node to node—a process termed **saltatory conduction**. The advantage of myelination is that it allows for rapid conduction while minimizing the metabolic demands on the cell. It also increases the packing capacity of the nervous system, so that many fast conducting fibres can be packed into a small nerve. As a result most axons over a certain diameter (~1 μm) are myelinated.

Disturbances in nerve conduction are clinically seen when there is a disruption of the myelin sheath, e.g. in the peripheral nervous system (PNS) in inflammatory demyelinating neuropathies such as the *Guillain–Barré syndrome* and in the central nervous system (CNS) with *multiple sclerosis* (see Chapter 59). In both conditions there is a loss of the myelin sheath, especially in the area adjacent to the node of Ranvier, which exposes other ion channels, as well as reducing the length of insulation along the axon. The result is that the propagated action potential has to depolarize a greater area of axolemma, part of which is not as excitable as the normal node of Ranvier because it contains fewer Na^+ channels. This leads to slowing of the action potential propagation and, if the demyelination is severe enough, actually leads to an attenuation of the propagated action potential to the point that it can no longer be conducted—so-called conduction block.

Synaptic integration

Each central neurone receives many hundreds of synapses and each input is integrated into a response by that neurone, a process that involves the summation of inputs from many different sites at any one time (**spatial summation**) as well as the summation of one or several inputs over time (**temporal summation**).

The presynaptic nerve terminal usually contains one neurotransmitter, although the release of two or more transmitters at a single presynaptic terminal has been described—a process termed **cotransmission** (see Chapter 9). The amount of neurotransmitter released is dependent not only on the degree to which the presynaptic terminal is depolarized, but also the rate of neurotransmitter synthesis, the presence of inhibitory presynaptic autoreceptors and presynaptic inputs from other neurones in the form of axoaxonic synapses (see Chapter 3). These synapses are usually inhibitory (presynaptic inhibition) and are more common in sensory pathways (see, for example, Chapter 20).

The released neurotransmitter acts on a specific protein or **receptor** in the postsynaptic membrane and in certain synapses on **presynaptic autoreceptors** (see Chapter 9). When this binding leads to an opening of ion channels with a cation influx in the postsynaptic process with depolarization, then the synapse is said to be **excitatory**, while those ion channels that allow postsynaptic anion influx or cation efflux with hyperpolarization are termed **inhibitory**.

Excitatory postsynaptic potentials (EPSPs) are the depolarizations recorded in the postsynaptic cell to a given excitatory synaptic input. The depolarizations associated with the EPSPs can go on to induce action potentials if they are summated in either time or space. **Spatial summation** involves the integration by the postsynaptic cell of several EPSPs at different synapses with the summed depolarization being sufficient to induce an action potential. **Temporal summation**, on the other hand, involves the summation of inputs in time such that each successive EPSP depolarizes the membrane still further until the threshold for action potential generation is reached. In contrast, **inhibitory postsynaptic potentials (IPSPs)** are hyperpolarizations of the postsynaptic membrane, usually as a result of an influx of Cl^- and an efflux of K^+ through their respective ion channels. IPSPs are very important in modulating the neurone's response to excitatory synaptic inputs (see figure). Therefore inhibitory synapses tend to be found in strategically important sites on the neurone—the proximal dendrite and soma—so that they can have profound effects on the input from large parts of the dendritic tree. In addition, some neurones can inhibit their own output by the use of axon collaterals and a local inhibitory interneurone (**feedback inhibition**), e.g. motorneurones and Renshaw cells of the spinal cord (see Chapter 36).

More **long-term modulations of synaptic transmission** are discussed in Chapters 39, 46 and 50, and in some disorders of the nervous system (e.g. epilepsy, multiple sclerosis) abnormal transmission of information may occur via non-synaptic mechanisms.

9 Neurotransmitters, receptors and their pathways

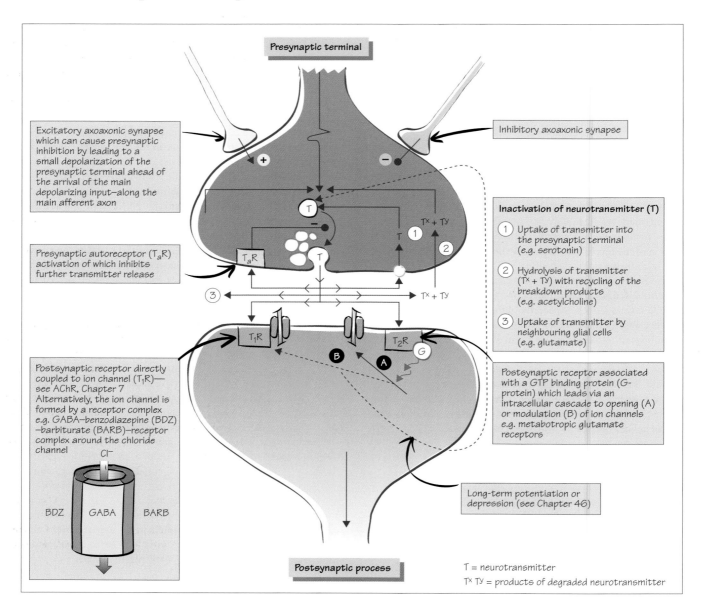

Presynaptic terminal

Excitatory axoaxonic synapse which can cause presynaptic inhibition by leading to a small depolarization of the presynaptic terminal ahead of the arrival of the main depolarizing input—along the main afferent axon

Inhibitory axoaxonic synapse

Presynaptic autoreceptor (T_aR) activation of which inhibits further transmitter release

Inactivation of neurotransmitter (T)

① Uptake of transmitter into the presynaptic terminal (e.g. serotonin)

② Hydrolysis of transmitter ($T^x + T^y$) with recycling of the breakdown products (e.g. acetylcholine)

③ Uptake of transmitter by neighbouring glial cells (e.g. glutamate)

Postsynaptic receptor directly coupled to ion channel (T_1R)—see AChR, Chapter 7 Alternatively, the ion channel is formed by a receptor complex e.g. GABA–benzodiazepine (BDZ) –barbiturate (BARB)–receptor complex around the chloride channel

Postsynaptic receptor associated with a GTP binding protein (G-protein) which leads via an intracellular cascade to opening (A) or modulation (B) of ion channels e.g. metabotropic glutamate receptors

Cl⁻

BDZ   GABA   BARB

Long-term potentiation or depression (see Chapter 46)

Postsynaptic process

T = neurotransmitter
T^x T^y = products of degraded neurotransmitter

Neurotransmitters and synaptic function

The neurotransmitter released at a synapse interacts with a specific protein in the postsynaptic membrane, known as a **receptor**. At some synapses the neurotransmitter also binds to a **presynaptic autoreceptor** that regulates the amount of transmitter that is released. Receptors are usually specific for a given neurotransmitter, although several different types of that receptor may exist. In some cases coreleased neurotransmitters can either modulate the binding of another neurotransmitter to its receptor or act synergistically on a common single ion channel (e.g. the **γ-aminobutyric acid (GABA)– benzodiazepine–barbiturate receptor**).

Receptors for specific neurotransmitters are either **coupled directly to ion channels** (T_1R on figure, e.g. acetylcholine receptors [AChR];

see Chapter 7) or **to a membrane enzyme (T_2R)**. In these latter instances the binding of the neurotransmitter to the receptor either opens an ion channel via an intracellular enzyme cascade (e.g. cyclic adenosine monophosphate [cAMP] and G-proteins) or indirectly modulates the probability of other ion channels opening in response to voltage changes (**neuromodulation**). These receptors therefore mediate slower synaptic events, unlike those receptors directly coupled to ion channels that relay fast synaptic information.

The activated receptor can only return to its resting state once the neurotransmitter has been removed either by a process of enzymatic **hydrolysis** or **uptake** into the presynaptic nerve terminal or neighbouring glial cells. Even then there are often intermediate steps in the process of returning the receptor and its associated ion channel to the resting state. At some synapses the affinity and, ultimately, the number of receptors is dependent on the previous activity of the synapse. For example, at catecholaminergic synapses the receptors become less sensitive to the released transmitter when the synapse is very active—a process of **desensitization and down-regulation**. This process involves a decrease in the affinity of the receptor for the transmitter in the short term, which goes on in the long term to an actual decrease in the number of receptors.

The converse is true with synapses that are rarely activated (**supersensitivity and up-regulation**), and in this way synaptic activity is modulated by its ongoing activity. In addition, at some synapses the activation of the postsynaptic receptor–ion channel complex can modulate the long-term activity of the synapse, either by affecting the presynaptic release of neurotransmitter or the postsynaptic receptor response—a process known as either **long-term potentiation (LTP) or long-term depression (LTD)** depending on the actual change in synaptic efficacy over time (see Chapters 39 and 46).

Therefore the state, number and types of receptors for a specific neurotransmitter as well as the presence of receptors to other neurotransmitters are all important in determining the extent of synaptic activity at any given synapse.

Diversity and anatomy of neurotransmitter pathways

The nervous system employs a large number of neurotransmitters, but these can be seen to form families (see Appendix 1).

Excitatory amino acids

These represent the main excitatory neurotransmitters in the central nervous system (CNS) and are important at most synapses in maintaining ongoing synaptic activity. The main excitatory amino acid is **glutamate** which acts at a number of receptors, which are defined by the agonists that activate them. The **ionotropic** receptors consist of the ***N*-methyl-D-aspartate (NMDA)** and **non-NMDA receptors**, and the former receptor with its associated calcium channel may be important in the generation of LTP (see Chapter 46), excitotoxic cell death (see Chapter 57) and possibly *epilepsy* (see Chapter 59).

A separate group of G-protein associated glutamate receptors, the **metabotropic receptors**, respond on activation by initiating a number of intracellular biochemical events that modulate synaptic transmission and neuronal activity. These receptors may underlie long-term depression in the hippocampus.

Inhibitory amino acids

The major CNS inhibitory neurotransmitters are **GABA**, which is present throughout the CNS, and **glycine** which is predominantly found in the spinal cord. Abnormalities of GABA neurones may underlie some forms of movement disorders as well as anxiety states and epilepsy (see Chapters 56 and 58) while mutations in the glycine receptor have now been linked to some forms of *hyperekplexia*—a condition in which there is an excessive startle response, such that any stimulus induces a stiffening of the body with collapse to the ground without any impairment of consciousness.

Monoamines

The monoaminergic systems of the CNS originate from small groups of neurones in the brainstem, which then project widely to all areas of the CNS. They are found at many other sites within the body, including the autonomic nervous system (see Chapter 16). In all locations they bind to a host of different receptors and thus can have complex actions including a role in depression, schizophrenia, cognition and movement control (see Chapters 40, 41, 48, 54 and 55).

Acetylcholine

This neurotransmitter is widely distributed throughout the nervous system, including the neuromuscular junction (see Chapter 7) and autonomic nervous system (see Chapter 16). Therefore, many agents have been developed that target the different cholinergic synapses in the periphery and which are used routinely in surgical anaesthesia. Several disease processes can affect the peripherally located cholinergic synapses (see Chapter 7), while secondary abnormalities in the central cholinergic pathways may be important in *Parkinson's disease and dementia of the Alzheimer type* (see Chapters 41 and 57).

Neuropeptides

These neurotransmitters, of which there are many different types, are found in all areas of the nervous system and are often coreleased with other neurotransmitters. They can act as conventional neurotransmitters as well as having a role in neuromodulation (e.g. pain pathways; see Chapters 23 and 24).

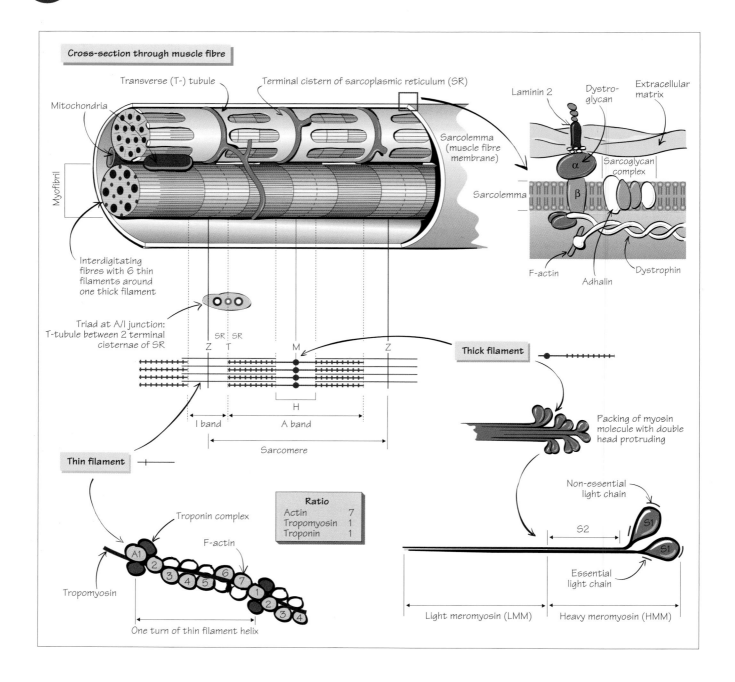

Skeletal muscle is responsible for converting the electrical impulse from a lower motorneurone that arrives at the neuromuscular junction (NMJ) into a mechanical force by means of contraction. The arrival of the action potential leads to the release of acetylcholine (ACh) which activates the nicotinic ACh receptor (AChR) in the postsynaptic muscle, which in turn leads to the depolarization of the muscle fibre (see Chapter 7). This produces a calcium influx into the muscle fibre which leads to muscle contraction (see Chapter 11).

Structure of skeletal muscle

Skeletal muscle is composed of groups of muscle fibres which are long, multinucleated cells. These fibres contain **myofibrils**, which in turn are made up of thick and thin filaments that overlap to some extent giving this type of muscle its striated appearance. The myofibrils are bounded by the **sarcolemma** which invaginates amongst the myofibrils in the form of **transverse or T-tubules**. This structure is separate from the **sarcoplasmic reticulum (SR)** which envelops the myofibrils and is important as an intracellular store of Ca^{2+}. The sarcolemma is a complex structure and abnormalities in some of its membrane components have recently been found to underlie some forms of inherited muscular dystrophies.

The **thick filament** is composed of myosin and lies at the centre of the **sarcomere**. Myosin is composed of two heavy chains that form the **light and heavy meromyosin proteins** (LMM and HMM, respectively). The HMM portion contains **S1 and S2 subfragments**. The S1 fragment consists of two heads and associated with each head are two light chains. The light chain found at the tip of the S1 head is termed **non-essential** and is responsible for breaking down adenosine triphosphate (ATP) at the end of the power stroke of crossbridge formation. The remaining **essential** light chain is attached at the point where the S1 head swings out towards the actin and is important in the process of myosin head movement. By virtue of the properties of LMM, myosin filaments spontaneously pack together so that the S1 heads are on the outside towards the actin filaments. The S1 heads therefore form the major part of the crossbridge with the actin.

Thin filaments are composed of **F-actin, tropomyosin and troponin**, which is itself composed of three subunits (troponin-I, -C and -T). These three components of the troponin complex all subserve different functions but as a whole they regulate muscle contraction by holding the tropomyosin in position so that it physically blocks the S1 head of the myosin from binding to the actin. The depolarization of the muscle leads to a calcium influx which then binds to troponin, producing a conformational change in the thin filament such that the tropomyosin shifts off the binding site for myosin on actin. Thus, tropomyosin and troponin regulate muscle contraction by a process of **stearic block**. In some muscles in other animals the regulation of the interaction between actin and myosin lies with the myosin-associated light chains.

At the point of overlap of these two sets of filaments the **triad** structure of a T-tubule linked to two terminal cisternae of SR by foot processes is to be found.

Disorders of structural proteins in skeletal muscle—the muscular dystrophies

There are many disorders of the muscle, which include disorders of excitability through mutations in the ion channels (see Chapter 5) as well as inflammation (see Chapter 59) and abnormalities in the structural proteins of the muscle itself. These latter conditions underlie many of the inherited muscular dystrophies of which the best characterized are Duchenne's and the limb girdle muscular dystrophies. ***Duchenne's muscular dystrophy (DMD)*** is an X-linked disorder in which there is a deletion of the gene coding for the structural protein dystrophin, with the milder form of the disease (***Becker's muscular dystrophy***) having a reduced amount of this same protein. Patients with DMD typically present early in life with clumsiness and difficulty in walking, with an associated wasting of the proximal limb muscles and pseudohypertrophy of the calf muscles. As the disease progresses the patient becomes increasingly disabled, with the development of cardiac and other abnormalities which lead to death, typically in the third decade. Characteristically, these patients have a raised creatine kinase (a marker of muscle damage) as the muscles in these patients are prone to necrosis as a result of the absence of dystrophin. This protein lies beneath the sarcolemma of skeletal (as well as smooth and cardiac) muscle and provides stability and flexibility to the muscle membrane, such that when absent the membrane can be easily disrupted. This allows entry of large quantities of Ca^{2+} which precipitates necrosis by excessive activation of proteases.

The ***limb girdle muscular dystrophies (LGMD)***, in contrast, can present at any age with progressive weakness of the proximal limb muscles and a raised creatine kinase. The condition can be inherited in a number of different ways, and recently the autosomal recessive forms of this condition have been found to contain abnormalities in the **dystrophin** associated glycoproteins, adhalin and the **sarcoglycan complex**. These proteins link the intracellular dystrophin with components of the extracellular matrix and so are important in maintaining the integrity of the sarcolemma.

Disorders with inflammation of skeletal muscle—the myositides

There are a number of disorders in which there is selective inflammation in skeletal muscle. This includes inflammation for unknown reasons with a predominant T-cell infiltrate (polymyositis); inflammation with a predominant B-cell mediated process (dermatomyositis) that can be paraneoplastic in nature; and a degenerative disorder that has a significant secondary inflammatory response (inclusion body myositis). The former two conditions tend to respond to immunotherapy, while inclusion body myositis does not. In all cases the inflammation damages the muscle, causing weakness often with pain, and a raised serum creatine kinase.

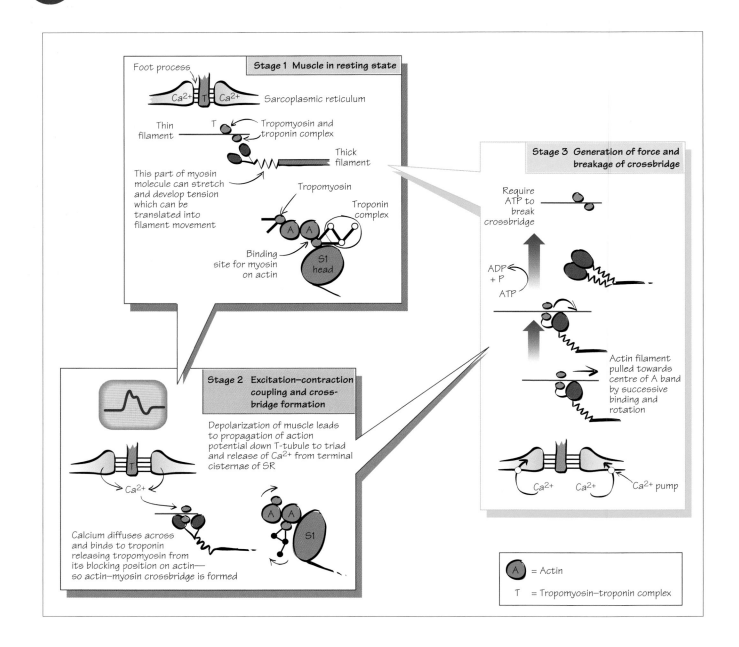

The arrival of the action potential at the neuromuscular junction (NMJ) leads to an influx of Ca^{2+} and the release of vesicles containing acetylcholine (ACh). This binds to the nicotinic ACh receptor (AChR) on the muscle fibre leading to its depolarization and Ca^{2+} release from the sarcoplasmic reticulum (SR) of the muscle. This leads to the removal of the blocking calcium-binding protein complex of **tropomyosin** and **troponin** from **actin**, the main component of the **thin filament**. The removal of this stearic block allows **myosin**, the major component of the **thick filaments**, to bind to actin via a **crossbridge**. The fibres are then pulled past each other; the crossbridge between the two fibres is broken at the end of this power stroke by the **hydrolysis of adenosine triphosphate (ATP)**. The cycle of crossbridge formation and breakage can then be repeated and the muscle contracts in a ratchet-like fashion.

The whole process is termed the **sliding filament hypothesis** of muscle contraction.

The sequence of events in the contraction of muscle is as follows.

• Stage 1: In the resting state the troponin complex holds the tropomyosin in such a position that it blocks myosin from binding to actin (stearic block).

• Stage 2: The arrival of an action potential at the NMJ causes a postsynaptic action potential to be initiated, which is propagated down the specialized invagination of the muscle membrane known as the **transverse tubule (T-tubule)**. This T-tubule conducts the action potential down into the muscle, so that all the muscle fibres can be activated. It lies adjacent to the terminal cisternae of the SR in a structure known as a **triad**, i.e. a T-tubule lies between two terminal cisternae of the SR (muscle equivalent of smooth endoplasmic reticulum) which contain high concentrations of Ca^{2+}. The T-tubules are linked to the SR by foot processes, which are part of a calcium ion channel. The arrival of the action potential at the triad leads to the release of Ca^{2+} from the terminal cisternae, by a process of mechanical coupling. The action potential opens a common Ca^{2+} ion channel between the T-tubule and SR, which then allows Ca^{2+} to influx down its electrochemical gradient towards the myofibrils. The Ca^{2+} then binds to the troponin complex and this leads to a rearrangement of the tropomyosin so that the myosin head can now bind to the actin, forming a crosslink or crossbridge.

• Stage 3: Once the myosin has bound to the actin there is a delay before tension develops in the crossbridge. The tension pulls and rotates the actin past the myosin and this causes the muscle to contract. The crossbridge at the end of this power stroke detaches the myosin from actin with hydrolysis of ATP, a process that is also calcium dependent. The whole cycle can then be repeated. The process of crossbridge formation with filament movement is called the **sliding filament hypothesis** of muscle contraction, as the two filaments slide past each other in a ratchet-like fashion as the cycle repeats. The Ca^{2+} released by the terminal cisternae of the SR, allowing the process of crossbridge formation and breakage, is actively taken back up into this structure by a specific Ca^{2+} pump.

Disorders of muscle contraction

Diseases of the muscles, which disrupt their anatomy, will lead to weakness as a consequence of a disorganization of contractile proteins. However, there are some disorders in which there is a disruption of the contractile process itself and examples of this are the rare *periodic paralyses* and *malignant hyperthermia/hyperpyrexia*. In this latter condition there is an abnormality in the ryanodine receptor which is part of the protein complex linking the T-tubule to the SR. This leads, under certain circumstances such as general anaesthesia, to sustained depolarization, contraction and necrosis of muscles resulting in an increase in body temperature and multiorgan dysfunction. In contrast, the *periodic paralyses* involve abnormalities in the ion channels that can lead to prolonged inexcitability of muscles, which thus become weak and paralysed. These are rare disorders and respiratory muscles are not involved; the paralysis can be provoked by a number of insults such as exercise or high carbohydrate meals.

It is also important to remember that disorders of muscle contraction occur as a consequence of abnormalities at the NMJ (see Chapter 7), as well as with some inborn errors of metabolism. These latter *metabolic myopathies* involve inherited defects in either carbohydrate or lipid metabolism which lead to either episodic exercise-induced symptoms or chronic progressive weakness.

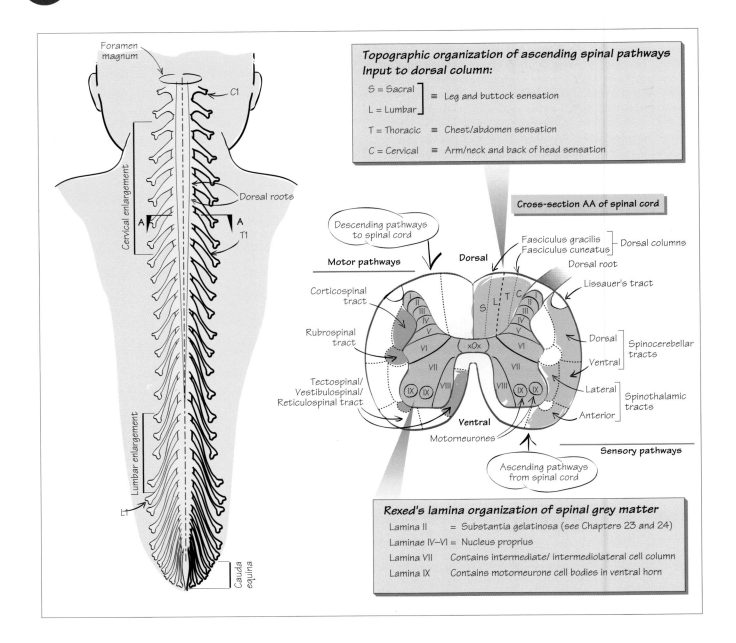

Topographic organization of ascending spinal pathways
Input to dorsal column:

S = Sacral] ≡ Leg and buttock sensation
L = Lumbar]

T = Thoracic ≡ Chest/abdomen sensation

C = Cervical ≡ Arm/neck and back of head sensation

Cross-section AA of spinal cord

Rexed's lamina organization of spinal grey matter
Lamina II = Substantia gelatinosa (see Chapters 23 and 24)
Laminae IV–VI = Nucleus proprius
Lamina VII Contains intermediate/ intermediolateral cell column
Lamina IX Contains motorneurone cell bodies in ventral horn

Overall structure

The spinal cord lies within the vertebral canal and extends from the foramen magnum to the lower border of the first lumbar vertebra; it is enlarged at two sites (cervical and lumbar regions) corresponding to the innervations of the upper and lower limbs (see Chapter 1). The lower part of the vertebral canal (below L1) contains the lower lumbar and sacral nerves and is known as the **cauda equina**.

Sensory nerve fibres enter the spinal cord via the **dorsal (posterior) roots** and their accompanying cell bodies are located in the dorsal root ganglia, while the motor and preganglionic autonomic fibres exit via the **ventral (or anterior) root**, together with some mostly unmyelinated afferent fibres. The **motor cell bodies (or motorneurones)** are found in the ventral horn of the spinal cord, while the preganglionic

cell bodies of the sympathetic nervous system are found in the **intermediolateral column** of the spinal cord.

The neuronal cell bodies that make up the central grey matter of the cord are organized into a series of **laminae (of Rexed)**. The white matter surrounding this is composed of myelinated and unmyelinated axons constituting the ascending and descending spinal tracts.

Organization of sensory afferent fibres entering the spinal cord

Sensory information from the peripheral receptors is relayed by primary afferent nerve fibres which terminate in layers I–V of the dorsal horn, the site for termination being different for different receptors. However, in reality, many afferent fibres divide (into an ascending

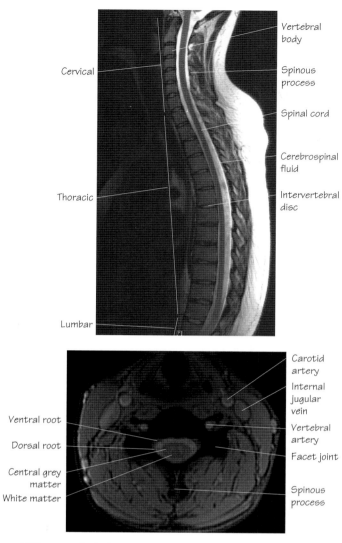

Cervical — Vertebral body

Spinous process

Spinal cord

Cerebrospinal fluid

Thoracic — Intervertebral disc

Lumbar

Ventral root — Carotid artery

Internal jugular vein

Dorsal root — Vertebral artery

Central grey matter — Facet joint

White matter

Spinous process

MRI scan of whole spine with a cross-sectional image of cervical spine.

and a descending branch) as they enter the spinal cord so that synaptic contact can be made both with many interneurones in the dorsal horn, and up and down the cord through Lissauer's tract.

Sensory processing in the dorsal horn

Typically, a number of primary afferents make synaptic contact with a single dorsal horn neurone. This **convergence** of input has the effect of reducing the acuity (accuracy) of stimulus location. However, the process of **lateral inhibition** helps minimize this loss of acuity by pro-

moting the inhibition of submaximally activated fibre inputs and thus increasing spatial contrast in the sensory input (see Chapter 20). The dorsal horn receives a number of descending inputs from supraspinal structures that are important in modulating the processing of sensory information through the spinal cord (see, for example, Chapter 23).

Ascending sensory pathways in spinal cord

The spinothalamic tract (STT), also known as the anterolateral system, spinocerebellar and dorsal columns (DCs) are the major ascending pathways of the spinal cord (see Appendix 2). Each tract relays specific information in a topographical fashion, i.e. the sensory information from different parts of the body is conserved in the organization of the ascending pathways. Inputs from the more rostral parts of the body (arm as opposed to leg) supply fibres that lie more laterally in the ascending pathway. Both the DC and STT **decussate** (fibres cross the midline) and therefore the sensory information they relay is ultimately processed in the **contralateral** cerebral hemisphere. However, the site at which this decussation occurs is different for the two pathways, with the anterolateral system crossing the midline in the spinal cord while the DCs decussate in the lower medulla after synapsing in the DC nuclei and forming the medial lemniscus (see Chapters 22 and 23).

Spinal motorneurones

α- and γ-motorneurones (MNs) are both found in the ventral (anterior) horn. The α-MN is one of the largest neurones found in the nervous system and innervates skeletal muscle fibres, while the γ-MN innervates the intrafusal muscle fibres of the muscle spindle (see Chapter 35). The cervical cord MNs innervate the arm muscles while the lumbar and sacral MNs innervate the leg musculature. The MNs are arranged **somatotopically** across the ventral horn such that the more medially placed MNs innervate proximal muscles, while those located more laterally innervate distal muscles (see Chapter 35).

Descending motor tracts

There are a number of descending motor pathways that are defined by their site of origin within the brain (see Appendix 2). The corticospinal (CoST) or pyramidal tract originates in the cerebral cortex and with the rubrospinal tract innervates the laterally placed MNs that supply the distal musculature. In contrast, the remainder of the extrapyramidal tracts (vestibulo-, reticulo- and tectospinal) innervate the more ventromedially placed MNs that control the axial musculature (see Chapters 34–38).

Clinical features of spinal cord damage
(see Chapters 33 and 43)
A knowledge of the organizational anatomy of the spinal cord allows one to predict the pattern of deficits with damage, which is of great value in clinical neurology. Examples of specific spinal cord lesions and syndromes illustrating this point are discussed in Chapters 33 and 43.

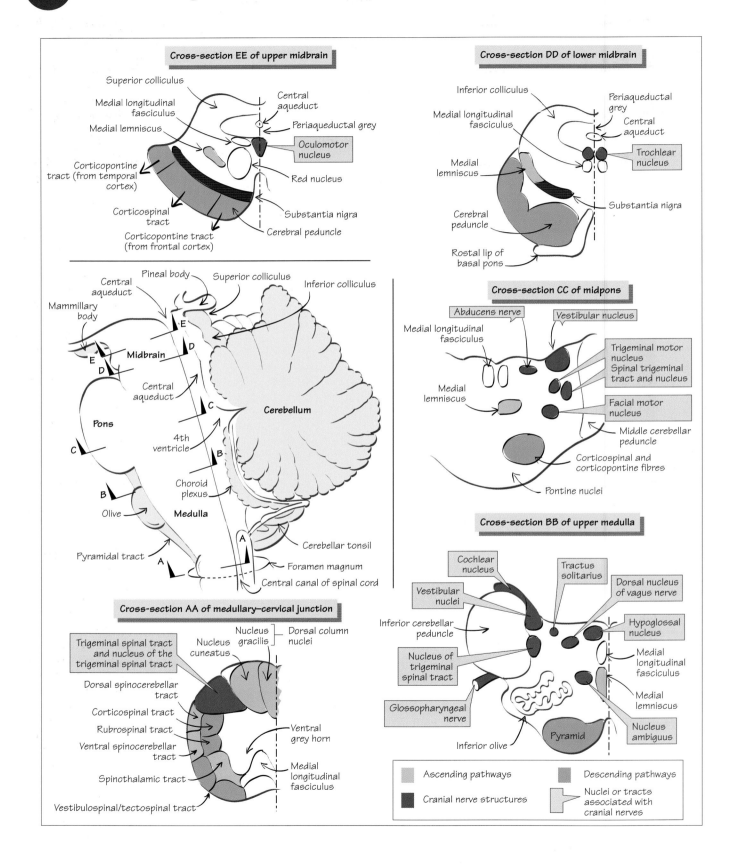

Cross-section EE of upper midbrain

- Superior colliculus
- Medial longitudinal fasciculus
- Medial lemniscus
- Corticopontine tract (from temporal cortex)
- Corticospinal tract
- Corticopontine tract (from frontal cortex)
- Central aqueduct
- Periaqueductal grey
- Oculomotor nucleus
- Red nucleus
- Substantia nigra
- Cerebral peduncle

Cross-section DD of lower midbrain

- Inferior colliculus
- Medial longitudinal fasciculus
- Medial lemniscus
- Cerebral peduncle
- Rostal lip of basal pons
- Periaqueductal grey
- Central aqueduct
- Trochlear nucleus
- Substantia nigra

- Central aqueduct
- Mammillary body
- Pineal body
- Superior colliculus
- Inferior colliculus
- E
- D
- **Midbrain**
- E
- D
- Central aqueduct
- **Pons**
- C
- C
- 4th ventricle
- **Cerebellum**
- Choroid plexus
- B
- B
- Olive
- **Medulla**
- Pyramidal tract
- A
- A
- Cerebellar tonsil
- Foramen magnum
- Central canal of spinal cord

Cross-section CC of midpons

- Abducens nerve
- Vestibular nucleus
- Medial longitudinal fasciculus
- Medial lemniscus
- Trigeminal motor nucleus
- Spinal trigeminal tract and nucleus
- Facial motor nucleus
- Middle cerebellar peduncle
- Corticospinal and corticopontine fibres
- Pontine nuclei

Cross-section BB of upper medulla

- Cochlear nucleus
- Vestibular nuclei
- Inferior cerebellar peduncle
- Nucleus of trigeminal spinal tract
- Glossopharyngeal nerve
- Inferior olive
- Tractus solitarius
- Dorsal nucleus of vagus nerve
- Hypoglossal nucleus
- Medial longitudinal fasciculus
- Medial lemniscus
- Nucleus ambiguus
- Pyramid

Cross-section AA of medullary–cervical junction

- Nucleus gracilis
- Nucleus cuneatus
- Dorsal column nuclei
- Trigeminal spinal tract and nucleus of the trigeminal spinal tract
- Dorsal spinocerebellar tract
- Corticospinal tract
- Rubrospinal tract
- Ventral spinocerebellar tract
- Spinothalamic tract
- Vestibulospinal/tectospinal tract
- Ventral grey horn
- Medial longitudinal fasciculus

Legend:
- Ascending pathways
- Cranial nerve structures
- Descending pathways
- Nuclei or tracts associated with cranial nerves

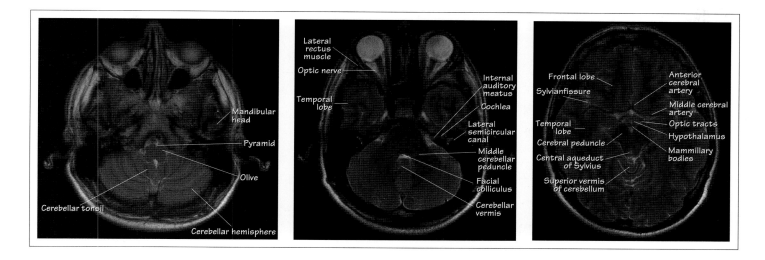

The brainstem consists of that part of the brain that begins at the **foramen magnum** and extends to the cerebral peduncles and thalamus. It consists of the **medulla, pons** and **midbrain** and is located anterior to the cerebellum to which it is connected by three cerebellar peduncles. It contains the following:

• The nuclei for 10 of the 12 pairs of **cranial nerves** (see Chapter 14), the exceptions being the olfactory and optic nerves.

• The apparatus for controlling eye movements which includes the third, fourth and sixth cranial nerves (see Chapter 42).

• The monoaminergic nuclei that project widely throughout the CNS (see Chapters 9, 24, 44 and 54)

• Areas that are vital in the control of respiration and the cardiovascular system, as well as the autonomic nervous system (see Chapter 16).

• Areas important in the control of consciousness including sleep, which include some of the monoaminergic nuclei (see Chapter 44).

• A number of ascending and descending pathways linking the spinal cord to supraspinal structures, such as the cerebral cortex and cerebellum, some of which take their origin from the brainstem (see Chapters 12, 20, 22–34, 36–39).

A number of structures found within the brainstem are worthy of special comment.

• The **dorsal column nuclei** represent the primary site of termination of the fibres conveyed in the dorsal columns (DCs), responsible for light touch, vibration perception and joint position sense. The relay neurones in this structure send axons that decussate in the lower medulla to form the **medial lemniscus** which synapses within the thalamus (see Chapter 22).

• The **pyramid** which represents the descending corticospinal tract (CoST) in the medulla, a pathway that decussates at the lower border of this structure.

• The **tractus solitarius** and **nucleus ambiguus** are associated with taste and the motor innervation of the pharynx by the glossopharyngeal and vagus nerves (see Chapter 14).

• The **inferior olive** in the medulla receives inputs from a number of sources and provides the climbing fibre input to the cerebellum (see Chapters 39 and 50).

• The **cerebellar peduncles** convey information to and from the cerebellum (see Chapter 39).

• The **medial longitudinal fasciculus** originates in the vestibular nucleus and projects rostrally connecting some of the oculomotor nuclei (third and sixth cranial nerves) as well as caudally to form part of the vestibulospinal tract.

• The **vestibular nucleus** has important connections from the balance organs within the inner ear and projects to the spinal cord and cerebellum as well as other brainstem structures (see Chapters 30, 36 and 39).

• The **substantia nigra** in the midbrain contains both dopamine and γ-aminobutyric acid (GABA) neurones, forms part of the basal ganglia and is involved in the control of movement (see Chapters 40–42). The loss of its dopaminergic neurones is the major pathological event in Parkinson's disease (see Chapter 41).

• The **red nucleus** in the midbrain is intimately associated with the cerebellum, and is the site of origin for the rubrospinal tract which, with the CoST, forms the lateral descending pathway of motor control (see Chapters 12, 35–38).

• The **periaqueductal grey matter** of the mesencephalon is an area rich in endogenous opioids and thus is important in the supraspinal modulation of nociception (see Chapter 23).

• The **central aqueduct of Sylvius** running through the midbrain connects the third to the fourth ventricle, and narrowing of it (stenosis) can cause hydrocephalus (see Chapter 18).

• The **cerebral peduncles** contain the descending motor pathways from the cerebral cortex to the spinal cord and brainstem, especially the pons (see Chapter 37).

• The **inferior colliculus** in the midbrain is part of the auditory system (see Chapter 29) while the **superior colliculus** is more involved with visual processing and eye movement control (see Chapters 26 and 42).

Thus, damage to the brainstem can have devastating consequences, although small lesions can often be localized with great accuracy because of the number of structures located within this small area of the brain. The most common causes of lesions in this part of the brain are either inflammatory (e.g. *multiple sclerosis*; see Chapter 59) or vascular in nature (see Chapter 19). However, disorders of the brainstem can also be seen with tumours (see Chapter 4) and a host of other conditions, and if damage is severe and extensive then it can be fatal. Testing specifically for brainstem functions is undertaken to assess if an individual with extensive brain injury (e.g. massive stroke or head injury) is brain dead, which has implications for further interventional therapy and organ donation. This assessment involves looking at reflex eye movements to head movement, eye movement responses to stimulation of the vestibular system and spontaneous respiration.

14 Cranial nerves

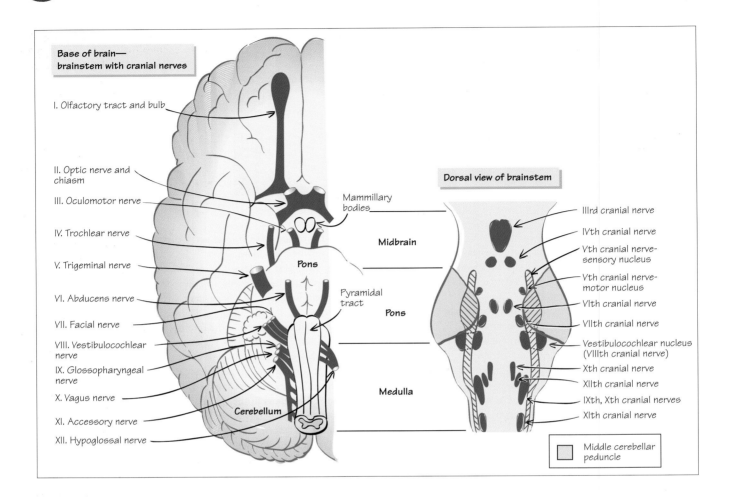

Base of brain—brainstem with cranial nerves

I. Olfactory tract and bulb
II. Optic nerve and chiasm
III. Oculomotor nerve
IV. Trochlear nerve
V. Trigeminal nerve
VI. Abducens nerve
VII. Facial nerve
VIII. Vestibulocochlear nerve
IX. Glossopharyngeal nerve
X. Vagus nerve
XI. Accessory nerve
XII. Hypoglossal nerve

Mammillary bodies
Midbrain
Pons
Pyramidal tract
Pons
Medulla
Cerebellum

Dorsal view of brainstem

IIIrd cranial nerve
IVth cranial nerve
Vth cranial nerve-sensory nucleus
Vth cranial nerve-motor nucleus
VIth cranial nerve
VIIth cranial nerve
Vestibulocochlear nucleus (VIIIth cranial nerve)
Xth cranial nerve
XIIth cranial nerve
IXth, Xth cranial nerves
XIth cranial nerve

Middle cerebellar peduncle

Cranial nerves

I Olfactory nerve

The receptors for olfaction are found within the nasal mucosa, and their axons project through the cribriform plate to the olfactory bulb on the undersurface of the frontal lobe (see Chapter 31). This cranial nerve therefore does not originate or pass through the brainstem, but is a central nervous system (CNS) structure and conveys information on smell. Damage to this nerve occurs most commonly with head trauma and shearing of the olfactory axons as they pass through the cribriform plate causing anosmia.

II Optic nerve

The photoreceptors in the eye project via bipolar cells to ganglion cells and then to the CNS via the optic nerve. The nerve passes through the optic canal at the back of the orbit into the brain and unites with the optic nerve from the other eye to form the optic chiasm. The fibres from here pass back as the optic tract to the lateral geniculate nucleus and from there as the optic radiation to the visual cortex (see Chapter 26). This cranial nerve therefore does not originate or pass through the brainstem, although it does have a projection to the midbrain which is important in controlling the **pupillary response to light** and some

reflex movement of the eyes (see Chapters 26 and 42), as well as to the hypothalamus which helps determine circadian rhythm.

Damage to this nerve will affect vision, although the extent and type of this visual loss is dependent on the site of injury (see Chapter 26)

III Oculomotor nerve

This originates in the midbrain at the level of the superior colliculus and supplies all the extraocular muscles apart from the lateral rectus which is supplied by the abducens (sixth cranial) nerve and superior oblique which is supplied by the trochlear (fourth cranial) nerve. The oculomotor nerve also carries the parasympathetic innervation to the eye as well as providing the major innervation of levator palpebrae superioris. A complete third nerve palsy causes the eye to lie 'down and out' with a fixed dilated unresponsive pupil and **ptosis** (droopy eyelid). Common causes of this are a posterior communicating artery aneurysm or a microvascular insult to the nerve itself as occurs in diabetes mellitus, for example.

IV Trochlear nerve

This nerve originates in the midbrain at the level of the inferior colliculus, and passes out of the brainstem dorsally. It supplies the superior oblique muscle and damage to this nerve causes double vision (diplopia) on looking down. A common cause of IV nerve palsy is head trauma.

V Fifth cranial or trigeminal nerve

The trigeminal nerve has both a motor and sensory function. The motor nucleus is situated at the midpontine level, medial to the main sensory nucleus of the trigeminal nerve, and receives an input from the motor cortex (see Chapter 37). It supplies the muscles of mastication. Sensation from the whole face (including the cornea) passes to the brainstem in the trigeminal nerve, and synapses in three major nuclear complexes: the nucleus of the spinal tract of the trigeminal nerve; the main sensory nucleus of the trigeminal nerve; and the mesencephalic nucleus. Sensation from the face is relayed via the three branches of the trigeminal nerve: the ophthalmic division that supplies the forehead; the maxillary division that supplies the cheek; and the mandibular branch that supplies the jaw—with the more rostral fibres (ophthalmic branch fibres) passing to the lowest part of the nucleus of the spinal tract in the upper cervical cord. These brainstem trigeminal nuclei in turn project to the thalamus as part of the somatosensory and pain systems (see Chapters 22–24). Damage to the trigeminal nerve results in weak jaw opening and chewing, coupled to facial sensory loss and an absent corneal reflex, and is usually caused by intrinsic lesions of the brainstem or damage to the branches as they pass out of the skull and cavernous sinus.

VI Sixth cranial or abducens nerve

This originates from the dorsal lower portion of the pons and supplies the lateral rectus muscle. Damage to it results in horizontal diplopia when looking to the lesioned side and can be caused by local brainstem pathology or can be a false localizing sign in raised intracranial pressure.

VII Seventh cranial or facial nerve

This is predominantly a motor nerve, although it does carry parasympathetic fibres to the lacrimal and salivary glands (via the greater superficial petrosal nerve and chorda tympani) as well as sensation from the anterior two-thirds of the tongue (via the chorda tympani). The motor nucleus for the facial nerve originates in the pons, and supplies all the muscles of the face except for those involved in mastication.

Damage to this nerve is not uncommon and can occur at any site along its long course, as it passes out of the brainstem through the internal auditory meatus, middle ear and mastoid and through the stylomastoid foramen and into the soft tissue structures of the face. A lesion of this nerve at any of these sites produces a lower facial nerve palsy with weakness of all the facial muscles ipsilateral to the side of the lesion. In addition, there is a loss of taste on the anterior two-thirds of the tongue if the lesion occurs proximal to the departure of the chorda tympani. This is most commonly seen in *Bell's palsy*. In contrast, damage to the descending motor input to the facial nucleus from the cortex (an upper motorneurone facial palsy) causes weakness of the lower part of the

contralateral face only, as the musculature of the upper part of the face has an upper motorneurone innervation from the motor cortex of both hemispheres (see Chapters 34, 36 and 43).

VIII Eighth cranial or vestibulocochlear nerve

This conveys information from the cochlea (the auditory or cochlear nerve; see Chapters 28 and 29) as well as the semicircular canals and otolith organs (the vestibular nerve; see Chapter 30). Damage to this nerve (e.g. in *acoustic neuromas*) causes disturbances in balance with deafness and tinnitus (a ringing noise).

IX Ninth cranial or glossopharyngeal nerve

The glossopharyngeal nerve contains motor, sensory and parasympathetic fibres. The motor fibres originate from the rostral nucleus ambiguus and supply the stylopharyngeus muscle, while the sensory fibres synapse in the tractus solitarius (or nucleus of the solitary tract) and provide taste and sensation from the posterior tongue and pharynx. The parasympathetic fibres originate in the inferior salivatory nucleus and provide an input to the parotid gland. Damage to this nerve is usually in conjunction with the vagus nerve (see below) and typically is seen with lesions in the lower brainstem and the skull base.

X Tenth cranial or vagus nerve

This nerve provides a motor input to the soft palate, pharynx and larynx, which originates in the dorsal motor nucleus of the vagus and nucleus ambiguus. It also has a minor sensory role, conveying taste from the epiglottis and sensation from the pinna, but has a significant parasympathetic role (see Chapter 16). Damage to the vagus nerve causes dysphagia and articulation disturbances and, as with glossopharyngeal nerve lesions, there may be a loss of the gag reflex. This reflex involves tongue retraction and elevation of the pharyngeal musculature in response to a sensory stimulus on the posterior pharynx.

XI Eleventh cranial or spinal accessory nerve

This is purely motor in nature and originates from the nucleus ambiguus in the medulla and the accessory nucleus in the upper cervical spinal cord and supplies the sternocleidomastoid and trapezius muscles. Damage to it causes weakness in these muscles, although in practice this nerve is usually damaged in conjunction with other lower cranial nerves.

XII Twelfth cranial or hypoglossal nerve

The hypoglossal nerve provides the motor innervation of the tongue. Its fibres originate from the hypoglossal nucleus in the posterior part of the medulla. Damage to this nerve causes wasting and weakness in the tongue which leads to problems of swallowing and speech, and is most commonly seen in *motorneurone disease* (see Chapter 57). Isolated damage of this nerve is rare and it is more commonly affected with other lower cranial nerves (e.g. IX, X, XI cranial nerves) and in such cases the patient may present with a *bulbar palsy*. A *pseudobulbar palsy*, in contrast, refers to a loss of the descending cortical input to these cranial nerve nuclei.

The organization of the cerebral cortex

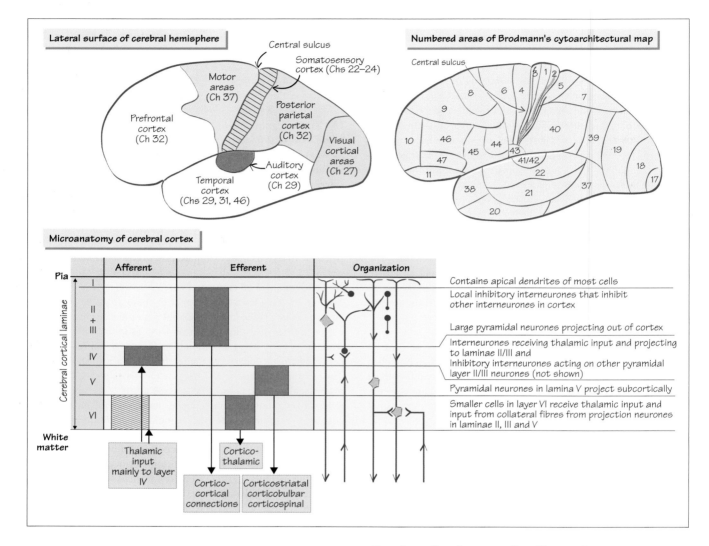

The organization of the outer layer of the cerebral hemisphere or **cerebral cortex** (neocortex) can be considered in various ways. Some of the earliest ways of doing this with cytoarchitectural maps are still used (e.g. **Brodmann's map** of the human brain from 1909). This way of mapping the cortex equates to some extent with the functional organization of this structure into motor, sensory and association areas, as evidenced by the **laminar organization** of the cortex. An area of cortex that is predominantly sensory in character has a prominent layer IV within it as this is the site of termination for thalamic afferent fibres, while cortical motor areas have a prominent layer V. An alternative approach is to view the cortex as being organized vertically. This vertical organization has become known as the **columnar hypothesis** and proposes that the 'column' of cortex is the basic unit of cortical processing and that the phylogenetic development of the cortex has involved an increase in the number of these columns. This explains why the enlargement of the neocortex in primates has been accomplished by a great expansion of its surface area, without striking changes in the number of neurones in a vertical penetration across the thickness of the cortex.

Anatomical organization of the cerebral cortex

The neocortex is classically described as consisting of six layers, although in certain areas of the cerebral cortex further subdivisions are used, e.g. the primary visual cortex (see Chapter 27). The thalamic afferent fibres, relaying sensory information, project to layer IV often with a smaller input to layer VI, and terminate in discrete patches thus ensuring that sensory information from a specific location and/or receptor type is relayed to a specific area of cortex. This input then synapses on interneurones within the cortex which in turn project vertically to neurones in layers II, III and V, which in turn project to other cortical and subcortical sites, respectively. Thus, the weight of synaptic relations within the cerebral cortex is in the vertical direction, although corticocortical connections linking columns of similar characteristics are found. This arrangement of synaptic connections is well seen in the somatosensory and visual cortices (see Chapters 22 and 27), and it means that a given sensory input from the thalamus will be analysed by a vertical column of cortical neurones. In cortical areas with a motor function, the motor output from that cortical area is such that it is directed back at the motorneurones (MNs) controlling the muscles that move the sensory receptors which ultimately project to that same area of cortex—so-called input–output coupling (see Chapter 37 for more details).

The anatomical evidence thus supports the notion of a vertical columnar organization to the neocortex, but further evidence comes from developmental and neurophysiological studies.

Developmental organization of the cerebral cortex

In the mammalian central nervous system (CNS) the entire population of cortical neurones is produced by a process of migration from the proliferative zones that are situated around the cavities of the cerebral ventricles. The **radial glial fibres**, which guide and may even give rise to the migrating neurones, span the fetal cerebral wall and direct the neurones to their correct cortical location in the developing **cortical plate** from the **ventricular and subventricular zones** (see Chapter 2). Thus, developmentally, the cortex forms in a vertical fashion.

Neurophysiological organization of the cerebral cortex

Neurophysiologically, if a recording electrode is passed at right angles through the cortex, it encounters cells with similar properties. However, if the electrode is passed tangentially then cells shift their response characteristics. This has been shown in all the primary sensory cortices, as well as the primary motor cortex (see Chapters 22, 27 and 38).

This columnar organization of the cortex means that topography can be maintained and that the reorganization of the cortex in the event of a change in the peripheral input is relatively straightforward (see Chapter 50).

Functional organization of the cerebral cortex

The relationship of cortical columns to one another raises many interesting questions as to the mode of function employed by the cerebral cortex. The original models on information processing in the cortex proposed that it was performed in a serial fashion, such that the cortical cells form a series of levels in a **hierarchy**. Thus, one set of cells perform a relatively straightforward analysis which then converges on another population of neurones that perform a more complex analysis (see, for example, Chapter 27). The ultimate prediction of these hierarchical models is that one neurone at the top of the hierarchy will register the percept—the **'grandmother' cell**. However, the discovery of the X, Y and W classes of ganglion cells in the retina (see Chapter 25) led to the development of a competing theory that proposed that information is analysed by a series of **parallel pathways**, with each pathway analysing one specific aspect of the sensory stimulus (e.g. colour or motion with visual stimuli; see Chapter 27). This theory does not exclude hierarchical processing but relegates it to the mode of analysis within separate parallel pathways. In practice, however, the cortex employs both modes of analysis.

It should be stressed that cortical columns are not to be viewed as a static mosaic structure, as one column may be a member of a number of different pathways of analysis. This organization has been termed the **distributed system theory** and describes the brain as a complex of widely and reciprocally interconnected systems, with the dynamic interplay of neural activity within and between these systems as the very essence of brain function. Consequently, one column may be a member of many distributed systems, because each distributed system is specific for one feature of a stimulus and one column may code for several features of the stimulus. An analogy for viewing this is to imagine the London underground system where each station is defined by the connections it has with other stations. Thus, one station may be part of many different lines, providing to each a unique quality. This analogy also helps explain the plasticity within the CNS, as damage to a station can be compensated for, up to a point, by the remaining networks as there is a degree of redundancy to the representation. However, if there is severe damage, especially of important centres or the peripheral terminals, then the system cannot compensate and lasting deficits ensue.

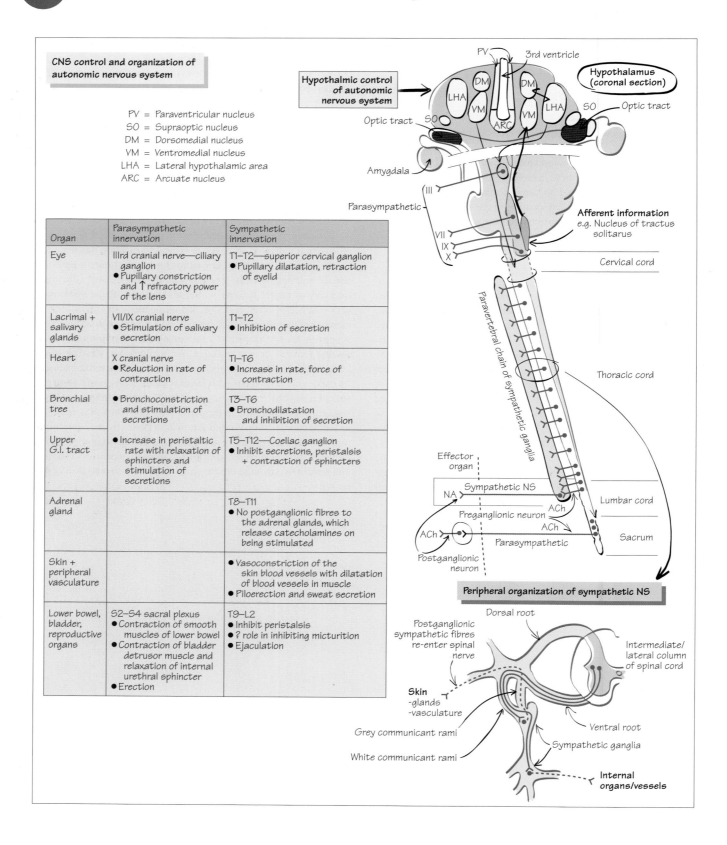

CNS control and organization of autonomic nervous system

PV = Paraventricular nucleus
SO = Supraoptic nucleus
DM = Dorsomedial nucleus
VM = Ventromedial nucleus
LHA = Lateral hypothalamic area
ARC = Arcuate nucleus

Hypothalmic control of autonomic nervous system

Hypothalamus (coronal section)

PV
3rd ventricle
DM
LHA
VM
ARC
SO
Optic tract
Optic tract
Amygdala

III
Parasympathetic

VII
IX
X

Afferent information
e.g. Nucleus of tractus solitarus

Cervical cord

Paravertebral chain of sympathetic ganglia

Thoracic cord

Effector organ

Sympathetic NS
NA
ACh
Preganglionic neuron

Lumbar cord

ACh
ACh
Parasympathetic
Postganglionic neuron

Sacrum

Peripheral organization of sympathetic NS

Dorsal root

Postganglionic sympathetic fibres re-enter spinal nerve

Intermediate/lateral column of spinal cord

Skin
-glands
-vasculature

Grey communicant rami

White communicant rami

Ventral root

Sympathetic ganglia

Internal organs/vessels

Organ	Parasympathetic innervation	Sympathetic innervation
Eye	IIIrd cranial nerve—ciliary ganglion • Pupillary constriction and ↑ refractory power of the lens	T1–T2—superior cervical ganglion • Pupillary dilatation, retraction of eyelid
Lacrimal + salivary glands	VII/IX cranial nerve • Stimulation of salivary secretion	T1–T2 • Inhibition of secretion
Heart	X cranial nerve • Reduction in rate of contraction	TI–T6 • Increase in rate, force of contraction
Bronchial tree	• Bronchoconstriction and stimulation of secretions	T3–T6 • Bronchodilatation and inhibition of secretion
Upper G.I. tract	• Increase in peristaltic rate with relaxation of sphincters and stimulation of secretions	T5–T12—Coeliac ganglion • Inhibit secretions, peristalsis + contraction of sphincters
Adrenal gland		T8–T11 • No postganglionic fibres to the adrenal glands, which release catecholamines on being stimulated
Skin + peripheral vasculature		• Vasoconstriction of the skin blood vessels with dilatation of blood vessels in muscle • Piloerection and sweat secretion
Lower bowel, bladder, reproductive organs	S2–S4 sacral plexus • Contraction of smooth muscles of lower bowel • Contraction of bladder detrusor muscle and relaxation of internal urethral sphincter • Erection	T9–L2 • Inhibit peristalsis • ? role in inhibiting micturition • Ejaculation

Anatomy of the autonomic nervous system

The **autonomic nervous system (ANS)** includes those nerve cells and fibres that innervate internal and glandular organs. They subserve the regulation of processes that usually are not under voluntary influence. The **efferent conducting pathway** from the central nervous system (CNS) to the innervated organ always consists of two succeeding neurones: one **preganglionic** and the other **postganglionic**, with the former having its cell body in the CNS (see Chapter 1).

The ANS is subdivided into the **enteric**, **sympathetic** and **parasympathetic nervous systems** with the latter two systems commonly exerting opposing influences on the structure they are both innervating. The sympathetic nervous system preganglionic neurones are found in the intermediate part (lateral horn) of the spinal cord from the upper thoracic to mid-lumbar cord (T1–L3). The preganglionic parasympathetic neurones have their cell bodies in the brainstem and sacrum. The postganglionic cell bodies are found in the vertebral and prevertebral ganglia in the sympathetic nervous system but in the parasympathetic system they are situated either adjacent to or in the walls of the organ they supply.

In addition to these anatomical differences there are pharmacological ones, with the sympathetic nervous system using **noradrenaline** (norepinephrine; NA) as its postganglionic transmitter while the parasympathetic nervous system uses **acetylcholine** (ACh). Both systems use ACh at the level of the ganglia.

Central nervous system control of the autonomic nervous system

The **CNS control of the ANS** is complex, involving a number of brainstem structures as well as the **hypothalamus** (see Chapter 17). The main hypothalamic areas involved in the control of the ANS are the ventromedial hypothalamic area in the case of the sympathetic nervous system and the lateral hypothalamic area in the parasympathetic nervous system. These controlling pathways can be direct or indirect via a number of brainstem structures such as the periaqueductal grey matter and parts of the reticular formation (see Chapter 13).

Clinical features of damage to the autonomic nervous system

Damage to the ANS can either be local to a given anatomical structure, or generalized when there is loss of the whole system caused by either a central or peripheral disease process. **Focal** peripheral lesions are not uncommon and the deficiencies resulting from these lesions can be easily predicted. For example, loss of the sympathetic innervation to the eye results in pupillary constriction (miosis), drooping of the upper eyelid (ptosis) and loss of sweating around the eye (anhydrosis)—a triad of signs known as *Horner's syndrome*. Other examples include the *reflex sympathetic dystrophies* where there is severe pain and autonomic changes confined to a single limb, often in response to some trivial injury (see Chapter 24). The exact role of the sympathetic nervous system in the genesis of these conditions is not known, as local sympathectomies are not always effective treatment and this condition has now been renamed *complex regional pain syndrome*. However, in some instances the nociceptors start expressing receptors for noradrenaline (norepinephrine; see Chapters 23 and 24).

More **global** damage to the ANS can occur because of degeneration of the central neurones either in isolation (e.g. *pure autonomic failure*) or as part of a more widespread degenerative process as is seen, for example, in *multiple-system atrophy* where there may be additional cell loss in the basal ganglia and cerebellum. Alternatively, the autonomic failure may result from a loss of the peripheral neurones, e.g. in diabetes mellitus, certain forms of amyloidosis, alcoholism and *Guillain–Barré syndrome*. Finally, abnormalities in the ANS can be seen with certain toxins (e.g. botulism; see Chapter 7) as well as in *Lambert–Eaton myasthenic syndrome* (LEMS; see Chapters 7 and 59).

In all these cases the patient presents with orthostatic and postprandial hypotension (syncopal or presyncopal symptoms on standing, exercising or eating a big meal) with a loss of variation in heart rate, bowel and bladder disturbances (urinary urgency, frequency and incontinence), impotence and loss of sweating and pupillary responses. The symptoms are often difficult to treat and a number of agents are employed to try to improve the postural hypotension and sphincter abnormalities. Such agents for postural hypotension include fludrocortisone, ephedrine, midodrine and vasopressin analogues (all of which cause fluid retention) and cisapride (a potentiator of ACh release) for the gastrointestinal paresis.

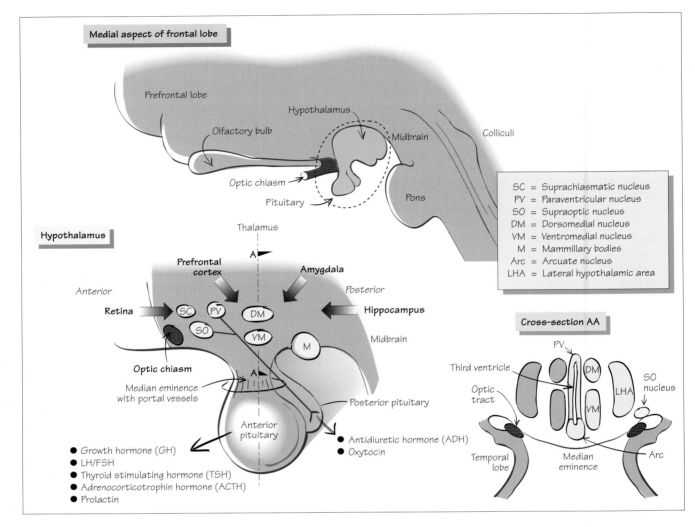

The hypothalamus lies on either side of the third ventricle, below the thalamus and between the optic chiasm and the midbrain, and receives a significant input from limbic system structures (see Chapter 46). It also receives from the retina, as well as containing a large number of neurones that are sensitive to changes in hormone levels, electrolyte changes and temperature changes. In addition to an efferent output to the autonomic nervous system (ANS), it has a critical role in the control of pituitary endocrine function (a detailed discussion on the endocrinology of the hypothalamic–pituitary system is beyond the scope of this book).

Thus, the hypothalamus, while being important in the control of the ANS, has a much greater role in the homoeostasis of many physiological systems (e.g. thirst, hunger, sodium and water balance, temperature regulation), the control of circadian and endocrine functions, the ability to form anterograde memories (in conjunction with the limbic system; see Chapter 46 and 47) and the translation of the response to emotional stimuli into endocrinological and autonomic responses.

The hypothalamus performs a number of other functions, all of which can be lost or deranged in the disease state. The most common cause is as a side-effect of surgical removal of ***pituitary tumours***.

The **functions of the hypothalamus** are as follows.
1 It controls the ANS and damage to it can cause autonomic instability. The ventromedial part of the hypothalamus has a major role in controlling the sympathetic nervous system while the lateral hypothalamic area controls the parasympathetic nervous system (see Chapter 16).
2 It controls the endocrine functions of the pituitary by the production of releasing and inhibiting hormones as well as producing antidiuretic hormone (ADH, also known as vasopressin) and oxytocin. Hypothalamic damage can have profound systemic effects because of the endocrinological disturbances associated with it, of which perhaps the most common example is neurogenic ***diabetes insipidus*** where there is loss of ADH. In this condition the patient passes many litres of urine each day, which needs to be compensated for by increased fluid intake. This is to be distinguished from nephrogenic diabetes insipidus where the problem lies within the ADH receptor in the kidney.
3 The hypothalamus has a major role in coordinating autonomic and endocrinological responses, both under physiologically appropriate conditions, and in the expression of emotional states as coded for by the limbic system. In cases of hypovolaemia or extreme anxiety, for example, the hypothalamus mediates not only increased sympathetic

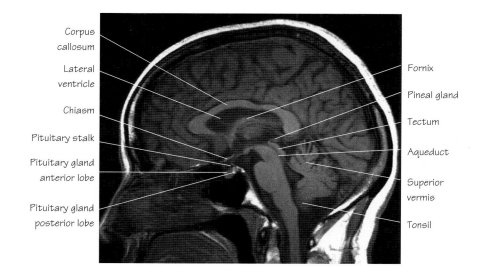

Corpus callosum
Lateral ventricle
Chiasm
Pituitary stalk
Pituitary gland anterior lobe
Pituitary gland posterior lobe

Fornix
Pineal gland
Tectum
Aqueduct
Superior vermis
Tonsil

activity, but also enhanced cortisol production via the stimulated release of adrenocorticotrophic hormone (ACTH) from the anterior pituitary. This is termed the stress response—which is defined by the rise in cortisol.

4 It has an important role in thermoregulation. Lesions to the anterior hypothalamic area cause hyperthermia, while stimulation of this same area lowers body temperature via the ANS, in contrast to the posterior hypothalamic area, which behaves in an opposite fashion. It may also mediate some of the more long-term changes seen with prolonged changes in ambient temperature, such as increased thyrotrophin-releasing hormone (TRH) production in patients exposed to a chronically cold enviroment. Damage to the hypothalamus can lead to profound changes in the central control of temperature. In septic states the production of some cytokines (e.g. interleukin-1) may reset the thermostat in the hypothalamus to a higher than normal temperature, accounting for the paradoxical situation of a fever with physiological evidence of mechanisms designed to conserve or generate heat (e.g. shivering).

5 It has a role in the control of feeding. In simple terms, the ventromedial hypothalamus is often called the satiety centre, in that damage to it causes excessive eating (hyperphagia) and weight gain, while damage to the lateral hypothalamic (or hunger) area produces aphagia (no eating at all). The control of these centres involves a number of hormones, including insulin and the more recently described leptins.

6 It has a role in the control of thirst and water balance by virtue of its osmoreceptors; the afferent input from a host of peripheral sensory receptors (e.g. atrial stretch receptors in the heart, arterial baroreceptors); the activation of hypothalamic hormone receptors (e.g. angiotensin II receptors); and its efferent output via the ANS to the heart and kidney as well as the production of ADH.

7 It has a role in the control of circadian rhythms via the retinal input to the suprachiasmatic nucleus. This nucleus appears to be critical in setting the circadian rhythm as lesion and transplant experiments have shown. Although the exact mechanism by which these rhythms are mediated is not known, it may involve the production of melatonin by the pineal gland.

8 It has a role with the limbic system in memory. Damage to the mammillary bodies, which receive a significant input from the hippocampal complex as occurs in chronic alcoholism with thiamine deficiency, produces a profound amnesia (***Korsakoff's syndrome***) of both an anterograde (inability to lay down new memories) and retrograde (inability to recover old memories) nature. The latter feature distinguishes these patients from those who have hippocampal damage (see Chapter 46 and 47) and may explain why patients with Korsakoff's syndrome tend to invent missing information (confabulation).

9 The hypothalamus may also have a role in sexual and emotional behaviour independent of its endocrinological influences.

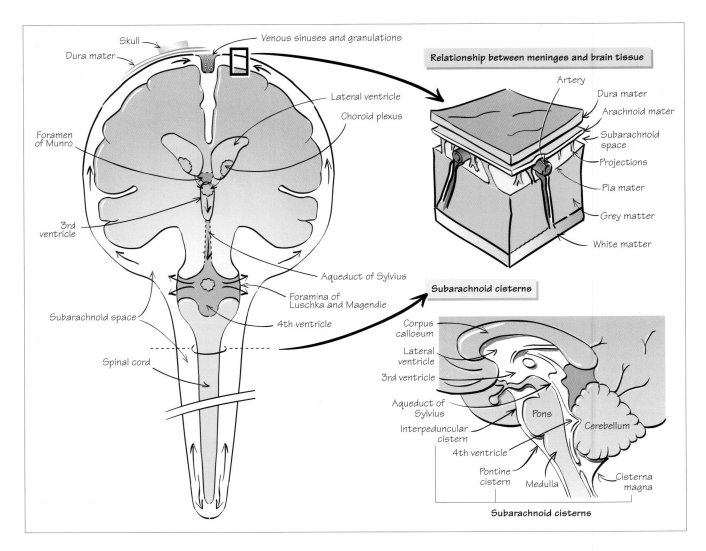

Cerebrospinal fluid production and circulation

Within the skull the brain is enclosed by three protective layers which also extend down the spinal cord. The **dura mater** is a thick tough membrane lying close to the skull and vertebrae and innervated by afferent fibres of the trigeminal nerve and upper cervical nerves. Headache can be associated with disturbance or inflammation of the dura. Adjacent to this is the **arachnoid mater**, a thin membrane with thread-like processes that project into the subarachnoid space and make contact with the delicate **pia mater** which envelopes the spinal cord and contours of the brain surface and dips into the sulci.

The **subarachnoid space** is filled with cerebrospinal fluid (CSF) and also accommodates major arteries, branches of which project down through the pia into the central nervous system (CNS). At specific sites the size of the subarachnoid space increases to form **cisterns**. These are particularly prevalent in the region of the brainstem and the largest is the **cisterna magna** found between the cerebellum and medulla.

The meninges extend caudally enclosing the spinal cord. Here the dura is attached to the foramen magnum at its upper limit and projects down to the second sacral vertebrae.

CSF is secreted by the **choroid plexuses** which are found primarily in the ventricles. The rate of production varies between about 300 and 500 mL/24 h and the ventricular volume is about 75 mL. CSF is similar to blood plasma although it contains less albumin and glucose. After production, CSF flows from the lateral ventricles into the third ventricle via the intraventricular foramina of Munro and then passes into the fourth ventricle via the central aqueduct of Sylvius and into the subarachnoid space via the foramina of Luschka and Magendie. From the subarachnoid space at the base of the brain CSF flows rostrally over the cerebral hemispheres or down into the spinal cord.

CSF reabsorption occurs within the superior sagittal and related venous sinuses. Arachnoid **granulations** are minute pouches of the arachnoid membrane projecting through the dura into the venous sinuses. The exact mechanism by which CSF is reabsorbed is not clear but does involve the movement of all CSF constituents into the venous blood.

As well as playing an important part in maintaining a constant intracerebral chemical environment (see below), the CSF also helps to protect the brain from mechanical damage by reducing the effect of impact damage experienced by the head.

Blood–brain barrier

The blood–brain barrier (BBB) used to be thought of as a single physical barrier preventing the passage of molecules and cells into the brain. More recently, however, it has been shown to be made up of a series of different transport systems for facilitating or restricting the movement of molecules across the blood–CSF interface. A characteristic of cerebral capillary endothelial cells is the presence of tight junctions between such cells, which are induced and maintained by astrocytic foot processes (see Chapter 4). These unusually tight junctions reduce opportunities for the movement of large molecules and cells, and thus require the existence of specific transport systems for the passage of certain critical molecules into the brain.

Small molecules such as glucose pass readily into the CSF despite not being lipid soluble. Larger protein molecules do not enter the brain but there are a number of carrier mechanisms that enable the transport of other sugars and some amino acids to occur. The effect of the barrier is to maintain a constant intracerebral chemical environment and protect against osmotic challenges, while granting the CNS relative immunological privilege by preventing cells from entering (see Chapter 59). However, from a therapeutic point of view the barrier reduces or prevents the delivery of many drugs (e.g. antibiotics) into the brain.

Clinical disorders

Hydrocephalus is defined as dilatation of the ventricular system and so can be seen in cases of cerebral atrophy, e.g. dementia (compensatory hydrocephalus). However, hydrocephalus can also occur as a result of increased pressure within the ventricular system, secondary to an obstruction in the flow of CSF (obstructive hydrocephalus). This typically occurs at the outlets from the fourth ventricle into the subarachnoid space, where the obstruction may be linked to the presence of a tumour, congenital malformation or the sequelae of a previous infection (see below). Alternatively, the flow of CSF from the third to the fourth ventricle may be impaired as a result of the development of *central aqueduct stenosis*. Hydrocephalus is also seen in rare conditions of oversecretion of CSF (e.g. tumours of the choroid plexus) as well as in the common situation of reduced absorption as occurs in *spina bifida*.

The symptomatology of hydrocephalus is varied but classically the patient presents with features of raised intracranial pressure (early morning headache, nausea, vomiting) and, in acute rises of pressure, altered levels of consciousness with brief periods of visual loss. Overall, probably the most common cause of raised intracranial pressure is a glial tumour (see Chapter 4) producing an effect by virtue of its mass, although such tumours in the posterior fossa can also directly cause hydrocephalus which may contribute to the raised intracranial pressure.

In obstructive hydrocephalus the treatment focuses on draining excess CSF using a variety of shunts linking the ventricles to either the heart (atrium) or the peritoneal cavity.

Meningitis

Meningitis or inflammation within the meningeal membrane can be caused by a number of different organisms. In acute infection there is the rapid spread of inflammation throughout the entire subarachnoid space of the brain and spinal cord, which produces the symptoms of headache, pyrexia, vomiting, neck stiffness (meningism) and, in severe forms of the disease, reduced levels of consciousness. The early administration of antibiotics is essential although the need to use and the type of antibiotic employed will depend on the nature of the organism responsible for the inflammation.

In other cases the infection or inflammation may follow a more subacute course, such as tuberculous meningitis or sarcoidosis. In cases such as this, secondary hydrocephalus may ensue as a result of meningeal thickening at the base of the brain obstructing CSF flow.

Rarely, tumours can spread up the meninges giving a *malignant meningitis*. This characteristically presents as an evolving cranial nerve or nerve root syndrome with pain. This is to be distinguished from primary tumours of the meninges—*meningiomas*—which are slow growing and benign and typically present with epileptic seizures or deficits secondary to compression of neighbouring CNS structures.

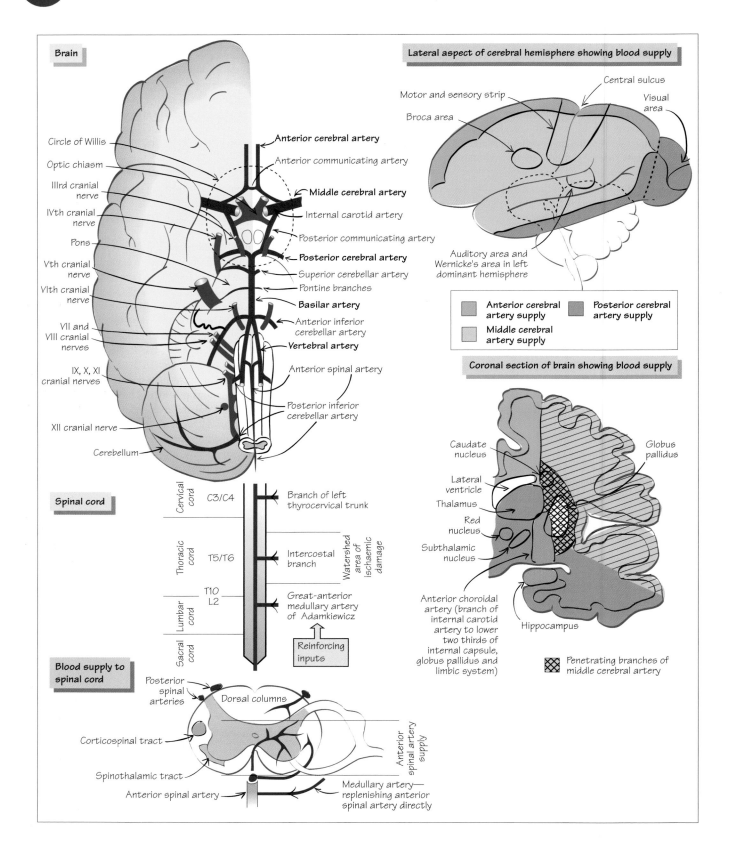

Brain

Circle of Willis
Optic chiasm
IIIrd cranial nerve
IVth cranial nerve
Pons
Vth cranial nerve
VIth cranial nerve
VII and VIII cranial nerves
IX, X, XI cranial nerves
XII cranial nerve
Cerebellum

Anterior cerebral artery
Anterior communicating artery
Middle cerebral artery
Internal carotid artery
Posterior communicating artery
Posterior cerebral artery
Superior cerebellar artery
Pontine branches
Basilar artery
Anterior inferior cerebellar artery
Vertebral artery
Anterior spinal artery
Posterior inferior cerebellar artery

Lateral aspect of cerebral hemisphere showing blood supply

Motor and sensory strip
Broca area
Central sulcus
Visual area
Auditory area and Wernicke's area in left dominant hemisphere

Anterior cerebral artery supply
Middle cerebral artery supply
Posterior cerebral artery supply

Coronal section of brain showing blood supply

Caudate nucleus
Lateral ventricle
Thalamus
Red nucleus
Subthalamic nucleus
Globus pallidus
Anterior choroidal artery (branch of internal carotid artery to lower two thirds of internal capsule, globus pallidus and limbic system)
Hippocampus
Penetrating branches of middle cerebral artery

Spinal cord

Cervical cord — C3/C4
Thoracic cord — T5/T6
Lumbar cord — T10 L2
Sacral cord

Branch of left thyrocervical trunk
Intercostal branch
Watershed area of ischaemic damage
Great-anterior medullary artery of Adamkiewicz
Reinforcing inputs

Blood supply to spinal cord

Posterior spinal arteries
Dorsal columns
Corticospinal tract
Spinothalamic tract
Anterior spinal artery
Anterior spinal artery supply
Medullary artery— replenishing anterior spinal artery directly

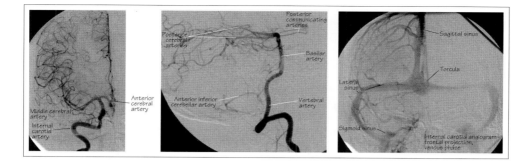

Blood supply to the brain

The arterial blood supply to the brain comes from four vessels: the right and left internal carotid and vertebral arteries. The **vertebral arteries** enter the skull through the foramen magnum and unite to supply blood to the brainstem (**basilar artery**) and posterior parts of the cerebral hemisphere (**posterior cerebral arteries**)—the whole network constituting the posterior circulation. The **internal carotid arteries (ICAs)** traverse the skull in the carotid canal and the cavernous sinus before piercing the dura and entering the middle cranial fossa just lateral to the optic chiasm. They then divide and supply blood to the anterior and middle parts of the cerebral hemispheres (**anterior and middle cerebral arteries; ACAs and MCAs,** respectively). In addition, the posterior and anterior cerebral circulations anastomose at the base of the brain in the **circle of Willis**, with the anterior and posterior communicating arteries offering the potential to maintain cerebral circulation in the event of a major arterial occlusion.

The **ICA** prior to its terminal bifurcation supplies branches to the pituitary (hypophysial arteries), the eye (ophthalmic artery), parts of the basal ganglia (globus pallidus) and limbic system (anterior choroidal artery) as well as providing the posterior communicating artery. The **MCA** forms one of the two terminal branches of the ICA and supplies the sensorimotor strip surrounding the central sulcus (with the exception of its medial extension which is supplied by the ACA) as well as the auditory and language cortical areas in the dominant (usually left) hemisphere. Therefore, occlusion of the MCA causes a contralateral paralysis that affects the arm and the lower part of the face and arm especially, with contralateral sensory loss or inattention and a loss of language if the dominant hemisphere is involved (see Chapters 22, 29, 33, 34, 37 and 38). In addition, there are a number of small penetrating branches of the MCA that supply subcortical structures such as the basal ganglia and internal capsule (see below).

The two **ACAs**, which form the other major terminal vessel of the ICA, are connected via the anterior communicating artery and supply blood to the medial portions of the frontal and parietal lobes as well as the corpus callosum. Occlusion of the ACA characteristically gives paresis of the contralateral leg with sensory loss, and on occasions deficits in gait and micturition with mental impairment and *dyspraxia* (see Chapters 22, 32, 33 and 43).

The **vertebral arteries**, which arise from the subclavian artery, ascend to the brainstem via foramina in the transverse processes of the upper cervical vertebrae. At the level of the lower part of the pons the vertebral arteries unite to form the **basilar artery** which then ascends before dividing into the two **posterior cerebral arteries (PCAs)** at the superior border of the pons. Each vertebral artery en route to forming the basilar artery has a number of branches including the posterior spinal artery, the posterior inferior cerebellar artery (PICA) and the anterior spinal artery. These spinal arteries supply the upper cervical cord (see below), whereas the PICA supplies the lateral part of the medulla and cerebellum. Occlusion of this vessel gives rise to the *lateral medullary syndrome of Wallenberg*.

The **PCAs** supply blood to the posterior parietal cortex, the occipital lobe and inferior parts of the temporal lobe. Occlusion of these vessels causes a visual field defect (usually a homonymous hemianopia with macular sparing, as this cortical area receives some supply from the MCA; see Chapter 26), amnesic syndromes (see Chapters 46 and 47), disorders of language (see Chapter 29) and, occasionally, complex visual perceptual abnormalities (see Chapter 27). The PCA has a number of central perforating or penetrating branches that supply the midbrain, thalamus, subthalamus, posterior internal capsule, optic radiation and cerebral peduncle. Are commonly affected in hypertension when their occlusion produces small **lacunar infarcts**.

Apart from occlusion, **haemorrhage** from cerebral vessels can occur which may be into the brain substance (intracerebral), the subarachnoid space or both. Such haemorrhages usually occur in the context of either trauma, hypertension or rupture of congenital aneurysms on the circle of Willis (*berry aneurysms*).

Venous drainage of the brain

Venous drainage of the brainstem and cerebellum is directly into the dural venous sinuses adjacent to the posterior cranial fossa. The cerebral hemispheres in contrast have internal and external veins—the external cerebral veins drain the cortex and empty into the superior sagittal sinus (see Chapter 18). This sinus drains into the transverse sinus, then the lateral sinus, before emptying into the internal jugular vein. The internal cerebral veins drain the deep structures of the cerebral hemisphere to the great vein of Galen and thence into the straight sinus. Occlusion of either of these venous systems can occur, causing raised intracranial pressure with or without focal deficits.

Blood supply to the spinal cord

The **blood supply to the spinal cord** comes in the form of a single anterior spinal artery and paired posterior spinal arteries. The anterior spinal artery arises from the vertebral arteries and extends from the level of the lower brainstem to the tip of the conus medullaris. The posterior spinal arteries take their origin from the vertebral arteries. At certain sites along the spinal cord there are a number of reinforcing inputs from other arteries (see figure).

Vascular insults to the spinal cord occur most commonly at the watershed areas in the cord, namely the lower cervical and lower thoracic cord. Occlusion of the anterior spinal artery produces a loss of power and spinothalamic sensory deficit with preservation of the dorsal column sensory modalities (joint position sense and vibration perception; see Chapter 33).

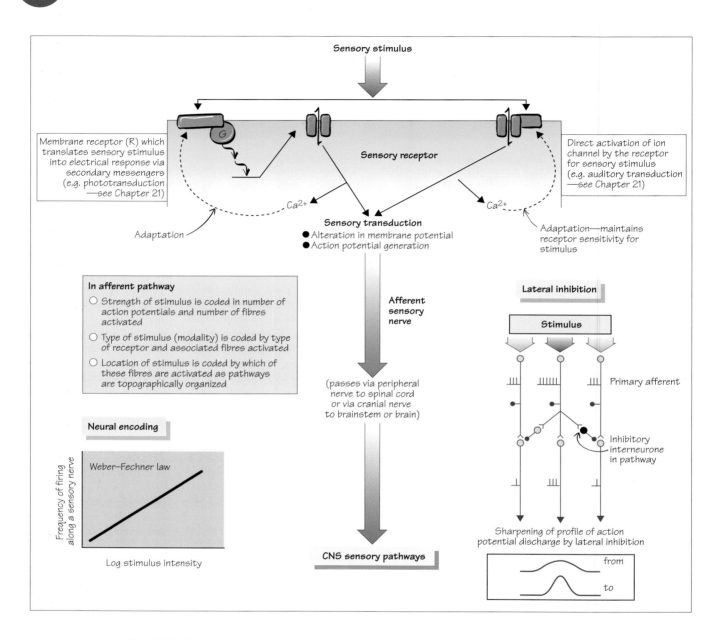

A sensory system is one in which information is conveyed to the spinal cord and brain from peripheral sensory receptors, which in themselves are either specialized neurones or nerve endings. The specialized **sensory receptor**, **afferent axon** and **cell body** together with the synaptic contacts in the spinal cord are known as the **primary afferent** and the process by which stimuli from the external environment are converted into electrical signals for transmission through the nervous system is known as **sensory transduction** (see Chapter 21). The signal produced by the sensory receptor is relayed to the central nervous system (CNS) via peripheral or cranial nerves and through a series of synapses eventually projects to a given area of cortex that is then capable of detailed analysis of that sensory input.

There are five main sensory systems in the mammalian nervous system: (i) touch/pressure, proprioception, temperature and pain or the somatosensory system (see Chapters 22–24); (ii) vision (see Chapters 25–27); (iii) hearing and balance (see Chapters 28–30); (iv) taste (see Chapter 31); and (v) smell or olfaction (see Chapter 31). All but the somatosensory pathways are regarded as 'special' senses.

Sensory receptors

Sensory receptors transduce the sensory stimulus either by a process of **direct ion channel activation** (e.g. the auditory system) or **indirectly via a secondary intracellular messenger network** (e.g. the visual system). In both cases the sensory stimulus is converted into an electrical signal that can then be relayed to the CNS in the form of either graded depolarizations/hyperpolarizations leading on to action potentials (e.g. visual system) or the direct generation of action potentials at the level of the receptor (e.g. auditory system; see Chapter 21).

The **specificity or modality** of a sensory system relies on the activation of specialized nerve cells or fibres which are highly specific for different forms of afferent stimuli, e.g. receptors in the retina are highly specific for photons although they may be activated by other stimuli in non-physiological circumstances such as pressure with compression of the eye. The receptor will only respond to stimuli when they are applied within a given region around it (its **receptive field**); an area of skin in the somatosensory system or a part of the retina in the case of photoreceptors, for example. This area or receptive field from which the receptor can be activated is recognized by the CNS as corresponding to a specific site or position in the body or outside world. However, the receptor will only transmit electrical information to the CNS when it receives a stimulus of sufficient intensity to reach the firing **threshold**. The incremental response to a change in stimulus intensity by the receptor gives the receptor its **sensitivity**. Many receptors have a high sensitivity both to the absolute level of stimulus detection and to changes in stimulus intensity because they are capable of both amplifying the original signal by the use of secondary messenger systems, and **adapting** to the presence of a continuous unchanging stimulus (see below and Chapter 21). Some receptors can change their sensitivity by altering the time and area over which they integrate incident stimuli, e.g. retinal rod photoreceptors in darkness. However, with very sensitive receptors the intrinsic instability of the transduction process is termed the **noise** and the challenge for the nervous system is to detect a sensory stimulus response or signal over this background noise (termed the **signal to noise ratio**).

The strength of a sensory stimulus can be coded for at the level of the receptor and its first synapse either in the form of action potentials or graded membrane potentials within the receptor which are subsequently converted into action potentials (see Chapter 21). The **afferent sensory nerve** can code (amongst other things) for the strength of the stimulus, first by increasing the number of afferent fibres activated (**recruitment or spatial coding**) and, secondly, by increasing the number of action potentials generated in each axon per unit time (**temporal or frequency coding**). However, the relationship between the stimulus strength and the number of action potentials generated is often non-linear because of the limited number of action potentials an axon can conduct by virtue of its refractory period (see Chapter 6). Thus, there is a more complex relationship between the stimulus intensity and action potential firing frequency in the afferent nerve—this is defined by the Weber–Fechner law.

The receptor, while being able to detect and code for the intensity of a specific sensory stimulus at a specific site, must also be capable of adapting so that it can respond to changes in the sensory information it receives. **Adaptation** is therefore defined as the decrease in receptor sensitivity that occurs in the presence of a maintained stimulus, and intracellular Ca^{2+} is an important mediator of this process in most sensory systems (see Chapter 21). If such a mechanism did not exist then a continuously applied stimulus would greatly reduce the sensitivity or even functionally 'inactivate' the receptor to any other new sensory inputs (e.g. the muscle spindle; see Chapter 35).

Sensory pathways

The coded information from the sensory receptors is relayed to the CNS via peripheral and cranial nerves, with each receptor having an associated axon. Each modality is associated with specific nerves or pathways, e.g. visual information is relayed via the optic nerve (see Chapter 26) while the somatosensory system relays information from a large number of peripheral nerves as well as the trigeminal nerve via the dorsal column–medial lemniscal system and spinothalamic tracts. Thus, each sensory pathway has its own unique input to the CNS, although ultimately most sensory pathways provide an input to the thalamus—the site of that projection being different for each sensory system. This in turn projects to the cortex, although the olfactory pathway primarily projects to limbic structures (see Chapter 31) and the muscle spindle to the cerebellum (see Chapter 39).

Each sensory system has its own area of cortex that is primarily concerned with analysing the sensory information and this area of cortex—the **primary sensory area**—is connected to adjacent cortical areas that perform more complex sensory processing (**secondary sensory areas**). This in turn projects into the **association areas** (posterior parietal, prefrontal and temporal cortices; see Chapter 32) which then project to the motor and limbic systems (see Chapters 34 and 46). These latter areas are more involved in the processing of sensory information as a cue for moving and generating complex behavioural responses.

The primary sensory cortical areas project not only to secondary sensory areas but also subcortically to their thalamic (and/or brainstem) projecting nuclei. This may be important in augmenting the detection of significant ascending sensory signals. This augmentation probably involves at least two major processes: **lateral inhibition** and **feature detection**. Lateral inhibition is a process by which those cells and axons with the greatest activity are highlighted by the inhibition of adjacent less active ones, which produces greater contrast in the afferent information. Feature detection, on the other hand, corresponds to the selective detection of given features of a sensory stimulus, which can occur at any level from the receptor to the cortex. Ultimately, the perception of any sensory stimulus relies on the synchronous activity of several areas of cerebral cortex (see Chapter 15).

Clinical disorders of the sensory pathways (see Chapter 33)

Damage at different sites in a sensory pathway produces a deficit, the extent and nature of which is dependent on the anatomical location. In general, the most devastating sensory losses are associated with damage to the receptors and their afferent pathways, while supraspinal lesions are often associated with more subtle deficits, which can be 'positive' in nature, e.g. paraesthesiae with focal *epilepsy* originating from the primary sensory cortex, or flashing lights with ischaemia of the visual cortex in *migraine*.

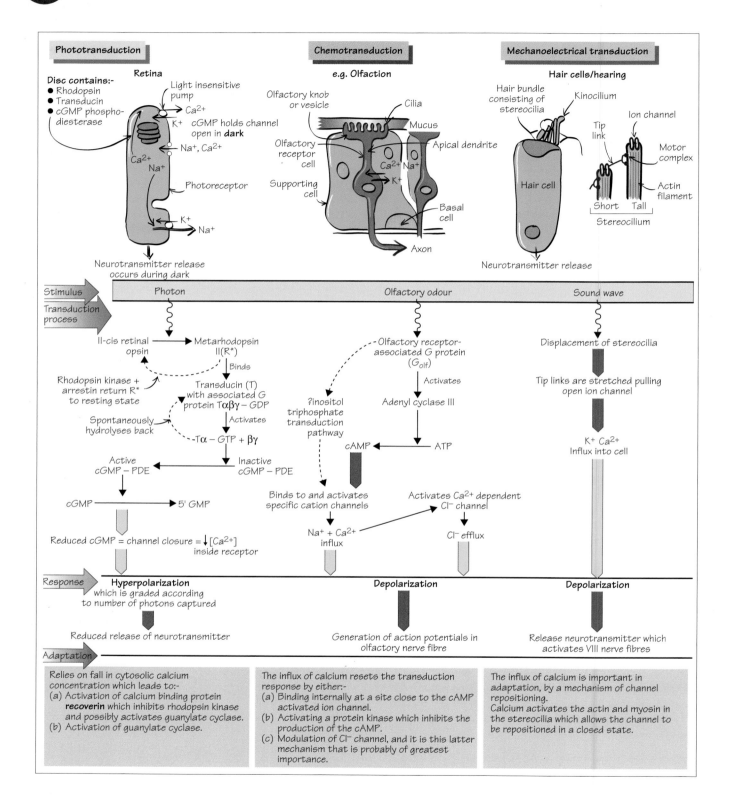

Sensory transduction involves the conversion of a stimulus from the external or internal environment into an electrical signal for transmission through the nervous system. This process is performed by all sensory systems and in general involves either a **chemical process** as occurs in the retina, tongue or olfactory epithelium, or a **mechanical process** as occurs in the cochlea and somatosensory systems. These contrasting modes of transduction are best characterized in some of the special senses.

Phototransduction

Phototransduction is the process by which light energy in the form of photons is translated into electrical energy in the form of potential changes in the photoreceptors (rods and cones) in the retina.

Photons are captured in pigments in the photoreceptor outer segment, which results in an amplification process using the G-protein, transducin and cyclic guanosine monophosphate (cGMP) as the secondary messenger. This results in reduced cGMP concentrations which leads to channel closure. The closure of these channels, which allow Na^+ and Ca^{2+} to enter the photoreceptor in the dark, leads to a hyperpolarization response, the degree of which is graded according to the number of photons captured by the photoreceptor pigment. The hyperpolarization response leads to reduced glutamate release by the photoreceptor on to bipolar and horizontal cells (see Chapter 25).

The termination of the photoreceptor response to a continuous unvarying light stimulus is multifactorial, but changes in intracellular Ca^{2+} concentration are important. The light insensitive Ca^{2+} pump in the outer segment coupled to the closure of the cation channel leads to a significant reduction in intracellular Ca^{2+} concentrations which is important in terminating the photoreceptor response as well as mediating light (or background) adaptation.

A number of rare congenital forms of **night blindness** have now been associated with specific deficits within the phototransduction pathway.

Olfactory transduction

Olfactory transduction is similarly a chemically mediated process. The olfactory receptor cells are bipolar neurones consisting of a dendrite with a dendritic knob on which are found the cilia, and an axonal part that projects as the olfactory nerve to the olfactory bulb on the underside of the frontal lobe. The presence of cilia, which contain the olfactory receptors, greatly increases the surface area of the olfactory neuroepithelium and so increases the probability of trapping odourant molecules. The binding of the odourant molecule to the receptor leads to the activation of G_{olf} which activates adenylate cyclase type III which hydrolyses adenosine triphosphate (ATP) to cyclic adenosine monophosphate (cAMP). cAMP then binds to and activates specific cation channels, thus allowing Na^+ and Ca^{2+} to influx down their concentration gradients. This not only partly depolarizes the receptor, but also leads to the activation of a Ca^{2+}-dependent Cl^- channel and the subsequent Cl^- efflux then further depolarizes the olfactory receptor. There are probably additional transduction processes present in the olfactory receptor using inositol triphosphate as the secondary messenger. This can lead to the generation of action potentials at the cell body which are then conducted down the olfactory nerve axons to the olfactory bulb.

The Ca^{2+} influx is also important in adaptation by resetting the transduction response.

Auditory transduction

In contrast to both phototransduction and olfactory transduction, the process of **auditory transduction** in the inner ear involves the mechanical displacement of stereocilia on the hair cells of the cochlea (see Chapter 28).

The sensory stimulus, a sound wave, causes displacement of the stapedial foot process in the oval window which generates waves in the perilymphatic filled scala vestibuli and tympani of the cochlea. This leads to displacement of the basilar membrane on which the hair cells are to be found in the organ of Corti. These cells transduce the sound waves into an electrical response by a process of mechanotransduction. The stereocilia at the apical end of the hair cell are linked at their tips by tip links, which are attached to ion channels.

The sound causes the stereocilia to be displaced in the direction of the largest stereocilia (or kinocilium) which creates tension within the tip links which then pull open an ion channel. This ion channel then allows K^+ (not Na^+, as the endolymph within the scala media is rich in K^+ and low in Na^+) and Ca^{2+} to flow into the hair cell and by so doing depolarize it. This depolarization leads to the release of neurotransmitter at the base of the hair cell which activates the afferent fibres of the cochlear nerve.

The continued displacement of the stereocilia in response to a sound is countered by a process of adaptation with a repositioning of the ion channel such that it is now shut in response to that degree of tip link tension. This is achieved by the influx of Ca^{2+} through the ion transduction channels which leads via actin-myosin in the stereocilia to a new repositioning of the ion channel in more of a shut state.

A number of syndromes with congenital deafness have now been identified as being caused by abnormalities in the myosin found in hair cells.

Other transduction processes

Transduction in the somatosensory receptors, nociceptors, thermoreceptors, taste receptors and muscle spindle are discussed in Chapters 22, 23, 31 and 35, respectively.

The somatosensory system

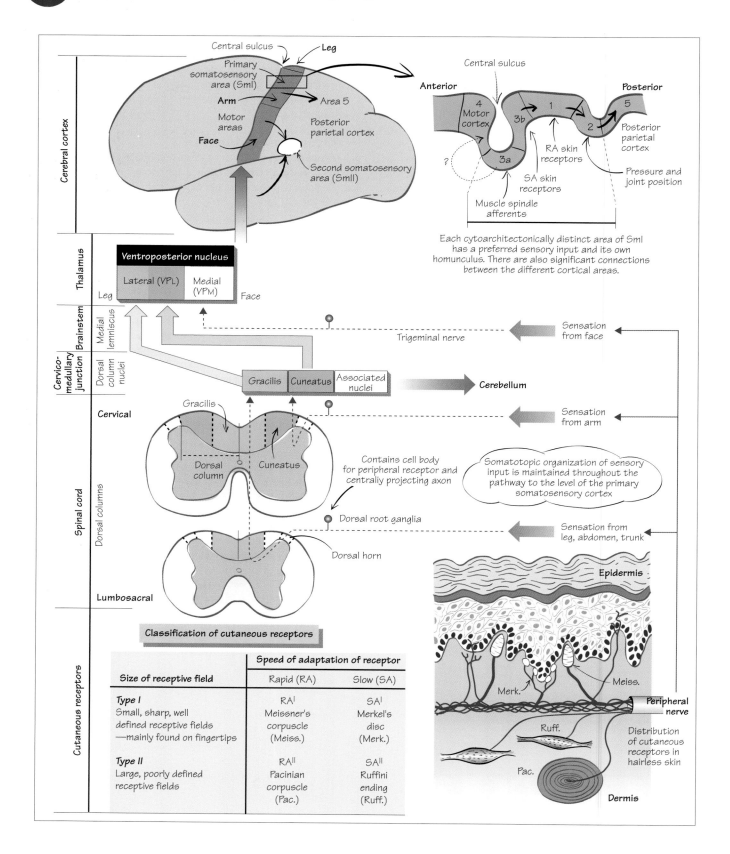

The somatosensory system is the part of the nervous system that is involved in the processes of touch, pressure, proprioception (or joint position sense; see also Chapter 35), pain and temperature perception (see Chapters 23 and 24).

Sensory receptors

The **receptors for touch** are specialized nerve endings located in the skin with their cell bodies in the dorsal root ganglia. They are found at particularly high density in the fingertips, while those for proprioception are found not only in the skin but also in the muscle and joints (see Chapter 35).

Skin receptors can best be characterized by their structure, location, receptive fields and speed of adaptation. Type I receptors with very small, sharply demarcated receptive fields (**Meissner's corpuscles** and **Merkel's discs**) are packed in high density at the fingertips and provide accurate information about the exact location of a felt stimulus. In contrast, the rapidly adapting (RA) **Pacinian corpuscles** convey vibration perception as they quickly stop firing to continuous sensory stimulus. The more slowly adapting (SA) **Ruffini endings**, on the other hand, sense the magnitude, direction and rate of change of tension in the skin and deeper tissues.

Dorsal column–medial lemniscal pathway

These receptors are specialized nerve endings and the fast conducting, large diameter axons associated with them are found in peripheral nerves and project into the **dorsal horn** of the spinal cord. The **trigeminal sensory system** for the face has a similar organization. Each class of receptor has a specific pattern of passage through the dorsal horn, but all ultimately end up in the **dorsal column** (with the exception of the trigeminal system), where they are organized according to receptor type and body location (somatotopy; see Chapter 12). They then project ipsilaterally up to the dorsal column nuclei at the cervicomedullary junction (consisting of the gracile and cuneate nuclei), where they make their first synapse, although it should be realized that many dorsal column axons synapse at other spinal sites.

The **dorsal column nuclei (DCN)** are a complex series of structures that lie at the cervicomedullary junction and send axons which immediately decussate to form the **medial lemniscus** which projects to the thalamus. The DCN also project to other brainstem structures, as well as receiving an input from the primary somatosensory cortex (SmI).

The medial lemniscus projects to the **ventroposterior (VP) nucleus of the thalamus**, picking up the trigeminal system as it ascends. This latter projection synapses in the medial part of the VP nucleus (VPM) with the remainder of the tract terminating in the lateral nucleus (VPL).

This medial lemniscal termination is in the form of an anteroposterior thalamic rod, where all the cells have a similar modality and peripheral location (e.g. index finger, RA type I receptors). The thalamic rod then projects to layer IV of the SmI and forms the basis of the cortical column (see also Chapter 15).

The **SmI** consists of four different areas (Brodmann's areas 3a, 3b, 1 and 2), each of which has a separate representation of the contralateral body surface, with the tongue being represented laterally and the feet medially. The cortical representation is proportional to the receptor density in the skin so, for example, the hand has a much greater representation than the trunk (the **sensory homunculus**).

Primary and secondary sensory cortices

Each cortical area within SmI has slightly different response properties with respect to the neurones found in these areas. As one moves posteriorly towards the posterior parietal cortex the response properties of the neurones become more complex, implying a higher level of cortical analysis. SmI projects not only back to the dorsal column nuclei but to the **posterior parietal cortex** and **second somatosensory area (SmII)**. This latter area is found in the lateral wall of the Sylvian sulcus and is important in tactile object recognition, while the posterior parietal cortex input from SmI is important in the attribution of significance to a sensory stimulus (see Chapter 32).

The primary somatosensory pathway has developed during evolution with the corticospinal tract (CoST), which has a selective role in the control of fine finger movements (see Chapters 36–38). These two systems act together in the process of 'active touch' by which we explore our environment. Both systems display a degree of plasticity even in adult life (see Chapters 37 and 50). This is in part made possible by somatotopic organization of the sensory pathway: adjacent areas of skin are represented in neighbouring parts of the sensory system, at least as far as SmI.

Clinical disorders of the somatosensory system

Damage to the receptors and their afferent fibres can occur in a large number of *peripheral neuropathies*. Patients typically complain of both paraesthesiae and numbness, often in association with alterations in proprioception especially if the dorsal root ganglion is involved (see Chapters 33 and 35).

Lesions to the dorsal columns in the spinal cord are described in Chapter 33. Damage to the somatosensory pathway above the level of the DCN produces a contralateral sensory loss that will involve the face if the lesion lies at or above the level of the upper brainstem.

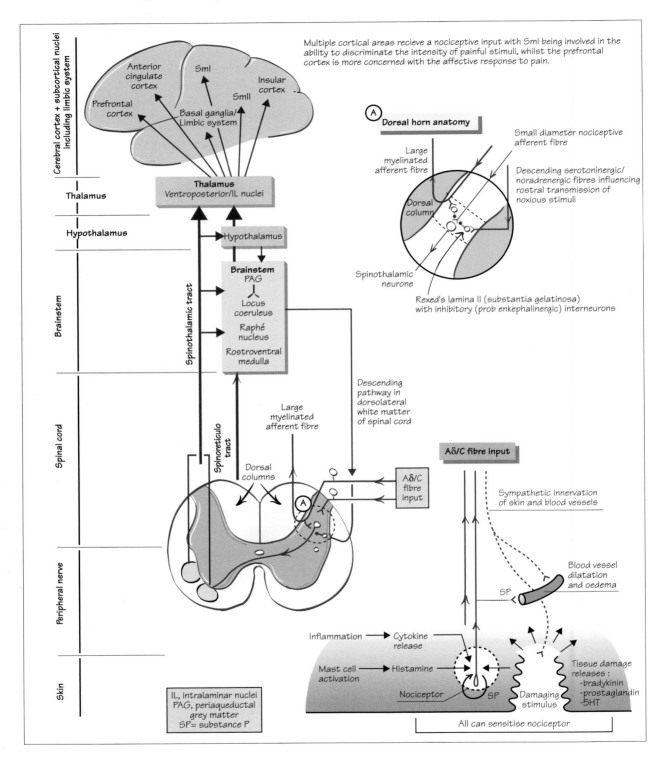

Multiple cortical areas recieve a nociceptive input with SmI being involved in the ability to discriminate the intensity of painful stimuli, whilst the prefrontal cortex is more concerned with the affective response to pain.

Pain is defined as an unpleasant sensory or emotional experience associated with actual or potential tissue damage or described in terms of such damage. Much of what is known about pain mechanisms has derived from animal-based research where the affective component is unclear and for this reason neuroscientists prefer to use the term **nociception** which defines the processing of information about damaging stimuli by the nervous system up to the point where perception occurs, at the level of the cerebral cortex and other subcortical structures. This is an important distinction because tissue damage is not inevitably linked to pain and vice versa.

Nociceptors

Nociceptors are found in the skin, visceral organs, skeletal and cardiac muscle and in association with blood vessels. They conduct information about noxious events to the dorsal horn of the spinal cord where the primary afferents synapse predominantly on interneurones.

There are basically two types of nociceptor, distinguished by the diameter of the afferent fibre and the stimulus required to activate it. The **high-threshold mechanoreceptor (HTM)** is activated by intense mechanical stimulation and innervated by **thinly myelinated Aδ fibres** conducting at 5–30 m/s. **Polymodal nociceptors (PMN)** respond to intense mechanical stimulation, temperatures in excess of about 42°C and irritant chemicals. These receptors are innervated by **unmyelinated C fibres** conducting at 0.5–2 m/s. Sharply localized pain is thought to be conducted in the faster conducting fibres whereas poorly localized pain is conducted in the C fibres.

Although nociceptors are histologically simple free nerve endings, the process of **transduction** at the receptor ending is complex and is associated with some of the chemical mediators of inflammation and tissue damage. Thus, adenosine triphosphate (ATP), bradykinin, histamine and prostaglandins all either activate or sensitize the receptor ending and indeed some of the transmitters in the nociceptive pathway are themselves released peripherally (e.g. substance P) to produce further sensitization of the receptor ending. Nociceptor receptor sensitization helps to explain the perception of heightened pain (**primary hyperalgesia**) in areas of tissue damage and is essentially a peripheral phenomenon and usually of relatively short duration.

Chronic and referred pain

Pain that lasts many months is known as chronic pain. It is often diasabling and resistant to treatment. It may arise following damage to either the peripheral or central nervous system or chronic inflammatory states (e.g., osteoarthritis). Changes in peripheral nociceptor sensitivity does not explain **secondary hyperalgesia** in which light touch outside the immediate area of cutaneous damage can lead to pain. A more serious problem associated with peripheral or central nerve damage is **allodynia**. In this condition light stroking of the skin can give rise to severe pain. Disturbed patterns of sensory input to the dorsal horn (e.g. following compression or sectioning of a peripheral nerve trunk) can lead to long-term changes in the processing of noxious information in the dorsal horn. At these sites, the arrival of axonally conducted substance P in the superficial layers of the dorsal horn leads to both an increase in receptive field sizes and the sensitivity of some dorsal horn neurones. These functional changes are mediated in part by the synaptic release of glutamate acting on postsynaptic *N*-methyl-D-aspartate (NMDA) receptors and may contribute to some chronic pain states.

In addition allodynia and secondary hyperanalgesia is also linked to increased activity in microglia and astrocytes and the release of a number of agents (interleukin-1 and -6, tumour necrosis factor [TNF], nitric oxide [NO], ATP and prostaglandins).

Damage to peripheral nerve trunks can lead to ***complex regional pain syndrome (CPRS)***. One form is associated with disturbances to the sympathetic nervous system (SNS) (CRPS-1, of which reflex sympathetic dystrophy is an example). Severing a peripheral nerve trunk leads to the formation of a neuroma which acts as generators of ectopic action potentials (ectopic foci) sending barrages of action potentials to the spinal cord. This activity is thought to explain the development of phantom limb pain with the neuroma being sensitive to both mechanical stimulation and SNS activity (ie, noradrenaline).

Visceral nociceptors project into the spinal cord via the small-diameter myelinated and unmyelinated fibres of the autonomic nervous system, and synapse at the spinal level of their embryological origin. The development of pain in an internal organ can therefore produce the perception of a painful stimulus in the skin rather than the organ itself, at least in the early stages of inflammation—a phenomenon known as referred pain. For example, inflammation of the appendix initially leads to pain being perceived at the umbilicus.

Nociceptive pathways

The majority of nociceptors and thermoreceptors project into the spinal cord via the dorsal root, although some pass through the ventral horn. On reaching the spinal cord these sensory nerves synapse in a complex fashion in the dorsal horn.

The postsynaptic cell conveying nociceptive information projects up the spinal cord as the **spinothalamic**, **spinoreticulothalamic** and **spinomesencephalic** tracts (latter not shown on figure), with the axons crossing at the spinal level by passing around the central canal of the cord. This crossing of fibres often occurs a few levels above where the nociceptive fibres enter the cord, and thus damage in the region of the central canal as occurs in *syringomyelia* leads to a loss of pain and temperature sensibility (see Chapter 33).

The postsynaptic cell and presynaptic nociceptive nerve terminal receive synapses from other peripherally projecting somatosensory systems, descending projections from the brainstem and interneurones intrinsic to the dorsal horn. Many of these interneurones contain **endogenous opioid substances** known as enkephalins and endorphins which activate opioid receptors of which there are three main subtypes (μ, κ, δ). There is therefore enormous potential for modifying the transfer of nociceptive information at the level of the dorsal horn (see Chapter 24).

The **ascending nociceptive pathways** synapse in a number of different central nervous system (CNS) sites. Information concerning noxious events ascends in either the spinothalamic tract (providing accurate localization) or the spinoreticulothalamic system (transmitting information concerning the affective components of pain). However, some of the nuclei in the brainstem to which these pathways project (e.g. the raphe nucleus and locus coeruleus) in turn send axons back down the spinal cord to the dorsal horn, and can be exploited in the control of chronic pain syndromes (see Chapter 24).

The thalamic termination of the spinothalamic pathway is in the ventroposterior and intralaminar nuclei (IL) (including the posterior group), which in turn project to multiple cortical areas but especially the primary somatosensory cortex (SmI) and second somatosensory area (SmII) and the anterior cingulate cortex. Lesions to any of these sites alter the perception of pain but do not produce a true and complete loss of pain or analgesia, and indeed may even produce a chronic pain syndrome. Such syndromes are not uncommonly seen with small thalamic cerebrovascular accidents.

The thermoreceptors, and to a lesser extent the nociceptors, also project to the hypothalamus which has an important role in thermoregulation, and the autonomic response to a painful stimulus (see Chapters 16 and 17).

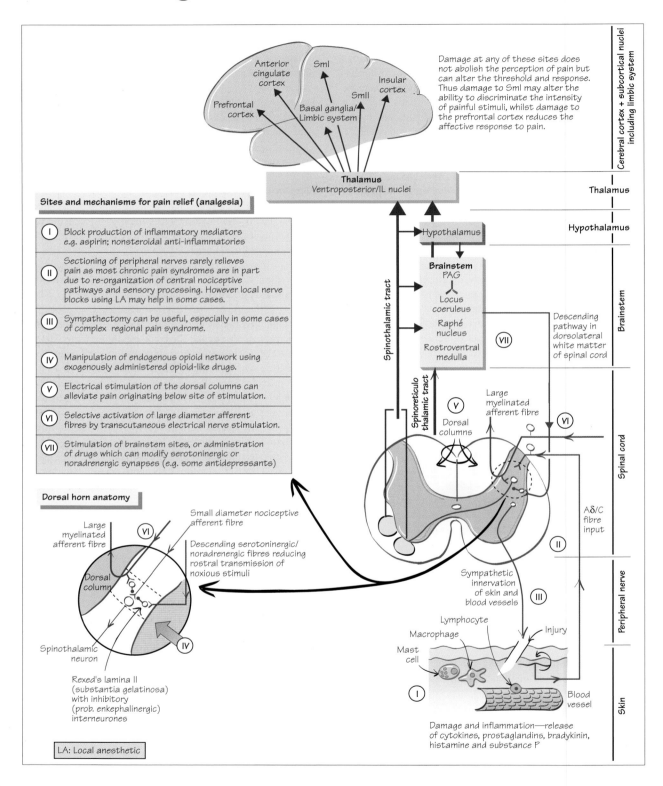

Damage at any of these sites does not abolish the perception of pain but can alter the threshold and response. Thus damage to SmI may alter the ability to discriminate the intensity of painful stimuli, whilst damage to the prefrontal cortex reduces the affective response to pain.

Cerebral cortex + subcortical nuclei including limbic system

Anterior cingulate cortex

SmI

Insular cortex

Prefrontal cortex

SmII

Basal ganglia/Limbic system

Thalamus
Ventroposterior/IL nuclei

Thalamus

Hypothalamus

Hypothalamus

Brainstem
PAG

Locus coeruleus

Raphé nucleus

Rostroventral medulla

Brainstem

VII

Descending pathway in dorsolateral white matter of spinal cord

Sites and mechanisms for pain relief (analgesia)

I — Block production of inflammatory mediators e.g. aspirin; nonsteroidal anti-inflammatories

II — Sectioning of peripheral nerves rarely relieves pain as most chronic pain syndromes are in part due to re-organization of central nociceptive pathways and sensory processing. However local nerve blocks using LA may help in some cases.

III — Sympathectomy can be useful, especially in some cases of complex regional pain syndrome.

IV — Manipulation of endogenous opioid network using exogenously administered opioid-like drugs.

V — Electrical stimulation of the dorsal columns can alleviate pain originating below site of stimulation.

VI — Selective activation of large diameter afferent fibres by transcutaneous electrical nerve stimulation.

VII — Stimulation of brainstem sites, or administration of drugs which can modify serotoninergic or noradrenergic synapses (e.g. some antidepressants)

Spinothalamic tract

Spinoreticulo thalamic tract

V — Dorsal columns

Large myelinated afferent fibre

VI

Spinal cord

Aδ/C fibre input

II

Dorsal horn anatomy

Large myelinated afferent fibre

VI

Small diameter nociceptive afferent fibre

Descending serotoninergic/noradrenergic fibres reducing rostral transmission of noxious stimuli

Dorsal column

IV

Spinothalamic neuron

Rexed's lamina II (substantia gelatinosa) with inhibitory (prob. enkephalinergic) interneurones

Sympathetic innervation of skin and blood vessels

III

Peripheral nerve

Lymphocyte

Macrophage

Mast cell

Injury

I

Blood vessel

Skin

Damage and inflammation—release of cytokines, prostaglandins, bradykinin, histamine and substance P

LA: Local anesthetic

The development of pain is a common experience and the treatment for it is important, not only where it is caused by injury or inflammation, but also in cases where the nerves themselves are damaged. In these latter cases the pain can arise from a site of previous injury (e.g. *allo-*

dynia) or may develop for more obscure reasons now renamed **complex regional pain syndrome**. In all cases the development of pain is both disabling and depressing and a multidisciplinary approach is often needed.

Management of pain

Pain relief or analgesia can be approached using a number of different strategies. Many analgesic therapies work by reducing the peripheral inflammatory response which is also responsible for receptor sensitization (**Site I** on figure).

Non-steroidal anti-inflammatory drugs (NSAIDs) are the most widely used analgesics. These drugs have analgesic, antipyretic and, at higher doses, anti-inflammatory actions. **Aspirin** was the first NSAID but has been largely replaced by drugs that are less toxic to the gastrointestinal tract, e.g. **paracetamol, ibuprofen, naproxen**. NSAIDs produce their effects by inhibiting **cyclo-oxygenase (COX)**, a key enzyme in the production of prostaglandins (PGs). PGs are one of the mediators released at sites of inflammation. They do not themselves cause pain but they potentiate the pain caused by other mediators, e.g. bradykinin, 5-HT, histamine (**Site I** on figure). NSAIDs are not effective in the treatment of visceral pain, which usually requires opioid analgesics. The most common adverse effects of NSAIDs involve the gut, e.g. dyspepsia, gastritis and, more seriously, gastrointestinal bleeding and perforation, and result from inhibition of PGs in the stomach. Newer NSAIDs (e.g. **valdecoxib**) selectively inhibit the isoform of cyclo-oxygenase involved in inflammation (COX-2) so have little effect on the constitutive isoform of the enzyme (COX-1) found in the gut but are associated with an increase in the incidence of myocardial infarction.

The interruption of peripheral nerve conduction by the injection of local anaesthetics can be helpful in some pain states, but lesioning of the peripheral nerve is usually without effect in ameliorating neuropathic pain (**Site II**). Unless it is to remove a neuroma in some cases.

The organization of the nociceptive input to the dorsal horn has been explored clinically in pain management. For example, stimulation of non-nociceptive receptors can inhibit the transmission of nociceptive information in the dorsal horn, which means that painful stimuli can be 'gated' out by counter irritation using non-painful stimuli. This is the basis of the **gate theory** of Wall and Melzack and is exploited clinically by the use of transcutaneous nerve stimulation (TENS) in areas of pain (**Site VI**), as well as the stimulation of the dorsal columns themselves in some cases of chronic pain (**Site V**). Similarly, the supraspinal input can also gate out noxious stimuli when activated (**Site VII**), as occurs in stressful situations when attending to a painful stimulus would not necessarily be useful (e.g. war injuries). These supraspinal nuclei can also be manipulated pharmacologically, with the administration of drugs that are normally used in the treatment of depression (see Chapter 54). These antidepressant drugs with a presumed action at the noradrenergic and serotoninergic synapse have been used to treat pain states, irrespective of any antidepressant action they might have (**Site VII**). The most commonly used agents are amine uptake inhibitors, such as imipramine and amitriptyline (tricyclic antidepressants). These agents appear to alter the pain threshold but are not without side-effects (see Chapter 59).

Furthermore, the recognition that one of the major transmitters in the nociceptive pathway is substance P (SP) has led to the development of other analgesic medications. For example, capsaicin (the active ingredient of red chilli), which initially releases SP from nociceptors and subsequently inactivates the SP-containing C fibres, can be used topically in some pain syndromes such as **postherpetic neuralgia**. However, perhaps the most common exploitation of this system medically is the manipulation of the enkephalinergic interneurone and opioid receptors by the exogenous administration of morphine and its analogues to control pain (**Site IV**).

Opioid analgesics are drugs that mimic endogenous opioid peptides by causing a prolonged activation of opioid receptors (usually µ-receptors). This reduces pain transmission at synapses in the dorsal horn of the spinal cord by an inhibitory action on the relay neurones. Opioids also stimulate noradrenergic, serotoninergic and enkephalinergic neurones in the brainstem that descend in the spinal cord and further inhibit the relay neurones of the spinothalamic tract. Opioid analgesics are widely used to relieve dull, poorly localized (visceral) pain. Repeated doses may cause dependence so that the sudden termination of opioid analgesics may precipitate a withdrawal syndrome.

Morphine is the most widely used analgesic in severe pain but, like all strong opioids, may cause nausea and vomiting. Other effects of morphine-type drugs include euphoria, respiratory depression, constipation and pinpoint pupils caused by stimulation of the third nerve nucleus.

Diamorphine (heroin) is more lipid soluble than morphine and therefore has a more rapid onset of action when given by injection and is widely used for postoperative pain.

Fentanyl can be given transdermally in patients with chronic stabilized pain. The patches are very useful in patients who suffer from intractable nausea or vomiting when taking oral opioids.

Methadone has a long duration of action and is less sedative than morphine. It is given orally for the maintenance treatment of heroin or morphine addicts. The methadone prevents the 'buzz' of intravenous drugs and so reduces the point of taking them.

Buprenorphine is a partial agonist at µ-receptors. It has a slow onset of action. It has a much longer duration of action than morphine (6–8 hours), but may cause prolonged vomiting.

Tramadol is a weak µ-agonist and its analgesic action is mainly a result of enhanced seronergic neurotransmission.

Codeine and **dextropropoxyphene** are weaker drugs used in mild to moderate pain.

Naloxone is an antagonist at opioid receptors and is used to reverse the effects of opioid overdose.

Although pain typically arises from tissue damage, it can also occur with damage to the peripheral (PNS) and central (CNS) nervous systems. One such example is trigeminal neuralgia, which is characterized by paroxysms of facial pain. In this condition the patient experiences paroxysms of pain in one of the three divisions of the trigeminal nerve and although in the majority of cases the cause of the condition is not found, it can be seen in some people with **multiple sclerosis**. It can be treated surgically by lesioning of the appropriate nerve root, although most cases respond to the antiepileptic agent **carbamazepine** or gabapentin (see Chapter 58). Another example of a pain syndrome arising with damage to neural tissue is seen following trauma to a peripheral nerve trunk, where a change in autonomic innervation to the traumatized limb results in the development of severe pain (see Chapter 23). The reason for the development of such states is not known, although the nociceptive nerve endings do appear to start expressing receptors for noradrenaline, so, local sympathectomies can be helpful in alleviating this pain, although this is not always the case (**Site III**).

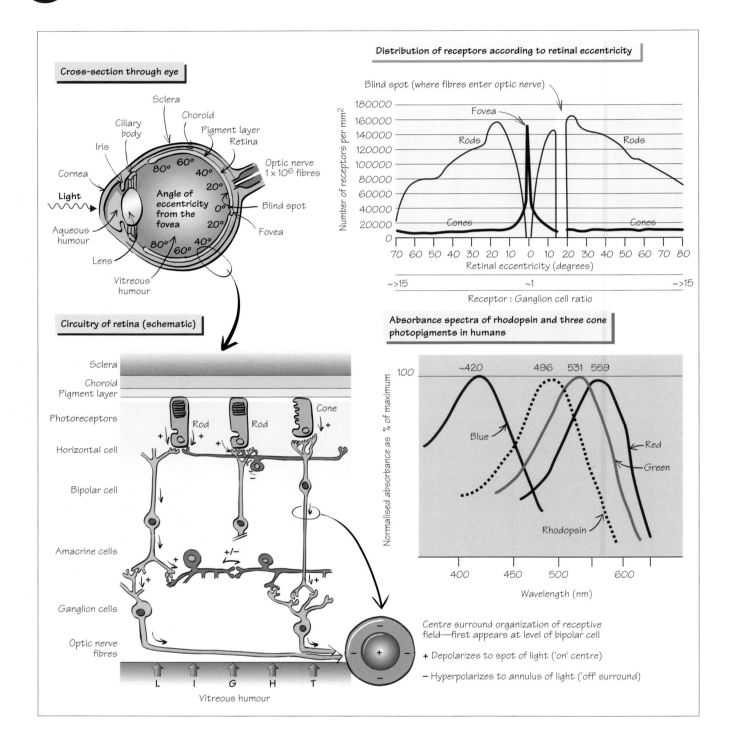

The visual system is responsible for converting all incident light energy into a visual image of the world. This information is coded for in the retina which lies at the back of the eye, and transmits that information to the visual cortical areas, the hypothalamus and upper brainstem (see Chapters 26 and 27). The process of visual transduction is detailed in Chapter 21.

Optical properties of the eye

On reaching the eye, light has to be precisely focused on to the retina, and this process of **refraction** is dependent on the curvature of the cornea and the axial length of the eye. Failure to do this accurately leads to an inability either to see clearly when reading (***long-sight or hypermetropia***), or to see distant objects clearly (***short-sight or*** *myopia*), or both. In the latter case there is often an additional problem of *astigmatism*, in which the refraction of the eye varies in different meridians.

In addition to the need to be refracted precisely on to the retina, light must also be transmitted without any loss of quality and this relies on the cornea, anterior and posterior chambers and lens all being clear. Injuries or disease of any of these components can lead to a reduced **visual acuity** (the ability to discriminate detail). The most common conditions affecting these parts of the eye are infections and damage to the cornea (*keratitis*) or opacification of the lens (*cataracts*).

Retinal anatomy and function

The light on striking the **retina** is transduced into electrical signals by the **photoreceptors** that lie on the innermost layer of the retina, furthest from the vitreous humour. There are two main types of photoreceptors: **rods and cones**. The rods are found in all areas of the retina, except the fovea; they are sensitive to low levels of light and are thus responsible for our vision at night (**scotopic vision**). Many rods relay their information to a single ganglion cell, and so this system is sensitive to absolute levels of illumination while not being capable of discriminating fine visual detail and colour. Thus, at night we can detect objects but not in any detail or colour.

The cones are found at highest density in the **fovea** and contain one of three different **photopigments**. They are responsible for our daytime or **photopic vision**. This, coupled to the high density of these receptors at the **fovea**, where they have an almost one-to-one relationship with ganglion cells, means that they are the receptors responsible for visual acuity and colour vision. Alterations in the photopigments contained within these receptors leads to *colour blindness*. Diseases of the receptors leading to their death, such as *retinitis pigmentosa*, lead to a progressive loss of vision that typically affects the peripheral retina and rods in the early stages, resulting in night blindness and constricted visual fields, although with time the disease process can spread to affect the cones.

The photoreceptors make synapses with both horizontal and bipolar cells. The **horizontal cells** have two major roles: (i) they create the centre surround organization of the receptive field of the bipolar cell; and (ii) they are responsible for shifting the spectral sensitivity of the bipolar cell to match the level of background illumination (part of the light adaptation response; see Chapter 21). The **centre surround receptive field** means that a bipolar cell will respond to a small spot of light in the middle of its receptive field in one way (depolarization or hyperpolarization), while an annulus or ring of light around that central spot of light will produce an opposite response. The horizontal cells, by receiving inputs from many receptors and synapsing on to the photoreceptor bipolar cell, can provide the necessary information for this receptive field to be generated. The mechanism by which they fulfil their other role in light adaptation is not fully understood.

The **bipolar cells** relay information from the photoreceptors to the ganglion cells and receive synapses from photoreceptors, horizontal and amacrine cells. They can be classified according to the receptor they receive from (cone only, rod only, or both) or their response to light. Bipolar cells that are hyperpolarized by a small spot of light in the centre of their receptive fields are termed **off-centre (on-surround)** while the converse is true for those bipolar cells that are depolarized by a small spot of light in the centre of their receptive field.

The **ganglion cells** are found closest to the vitreous humour, receive from both bipolar and amacrine cells and send their axons to the brain via the optic nerve. These nerve fibres course over the inner surface of the retina before leaving at a site which forms the **optic disc** and which is responsible for the **blind spot** as no receptors are located at this site. This blind spot is not usually apparent in normal vision. The ganglion cells can be classified in a number of different ways: according to their morphology; their response to light as for bipolar cells ('on' or 'off' centre); or a combination of these properties (the **XYW system in cats** or **the M and P channels in primates**). The X ganglion cells, which make up 80% of the retinal ganglion cell population, are involved in the analysis of detail and colour while the Y ganglion cells are more involved in motion detection. The W ganglion cells, which make up the remaining 10% of the population, project to the brainstem but as yet have no clearly defined function. The X and Y ganglion cell system defined initially in cats is equivalent to the P and M channel in primates, which is broadly responsible for 'form' and 'movement' coding, respectively. In addition, there is a small population of ganglion cells that contain a protein called melanopsin which allows them to detect light independently of photoreceptors. These ganglion cells project to multiple sites within the CNS but especially the suprachiasmatic nucleus of the hypothalamus (see Chapters 17 and 26)

The **amacrine cells** of the retina, which make up the final class of retinal cells, receive and relay signals from and to bipolar cells, other amacrine cells and ganglion cells. There are many different types of amacrine cells, some of which are exclusively related to rods and others to cones, and they contain a number of different transmitters. They tend to have complex responses to light stimuli and are important in generating many of the response properties of ganglion cells, including the detection and coding of moving objects and the onset and offset of illumination.

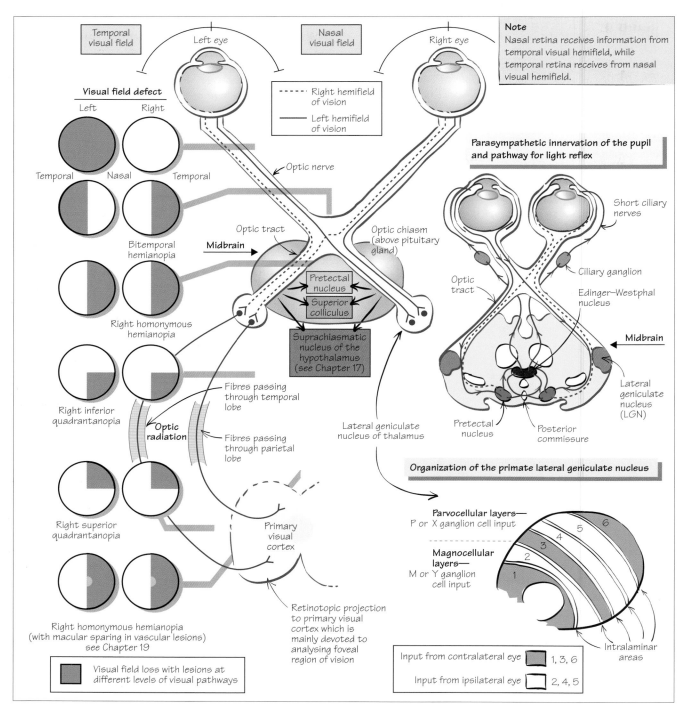

The **retina** conveys its information from the ganglion cells to a number of different sites, including several cortical areas, via the thalamus, the hypothalamus and midbrain. The major cortical projection is via the lateral geniculate nucleus (LGN) of the thalamus to the primary visual cortex (V1 or Brodmann's area 17). Other cortical areas (known collectively as the extrastriate areas) receive information from the LGN as well as the pulvinar region of the thalamus (see Chapter 27).

The projection from the retina to V1 maintains its retinotopic organization, such that a lesion along the course of the pathway produces a predictable visual field defect. Lesions in front of the optic chiasm typically produce uniocular field defects while lesions of the chiasm (e.g. from pituitary tumours) cause a bitemporal hemianopia. Lesions behind the chiasm typically produce similar field defects in both eyes, e.g. a homonymous hemianopia or quandrantanopia.

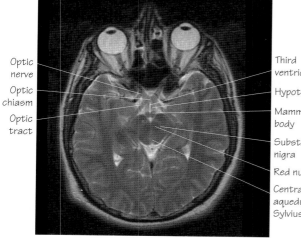

Optic nerve
Optic chiasm
Optic tract
Third ventricle
Hypothalamus
Mammillary body
Substantia nigra
Red nucleus
Central aqueduct of Sylvius

Superior colliculus

The superior colliculus in the midbrain is a multilayered structure, wherein the superficial layers are involved in mapping the visual field and the deep layers with complex sensory integration involving visual, auditory and somatosensory stimuli. The intermediate layers are involved in saccadic eye movements and receive connections from the occipitoparietal cortex, the frontal eye fields and the substantia nigra (see Chapter 42). The saccadic eye movements are tightly mapped in the superior colliculus, so that stimulation at a given point within it will cause a saccadic eye movement to bring the point of fixation to that point in the visual field that is represented in the more superficial layers of this structure. This ability to line up different sensorimotor representations in the superior colliculus in register even extends down into the deeper layers. In other words, a vertical descent through this structure encounters, in order: (i) neurones that respond to visual stimuli in a given part of the visual field; (ii) neurones that cause saccadic eye movements that bring the fovea to bear on to that same part of the visual scene; (iii) auditory and somatosensory neurones that are maximally activated by sounds that originate from that part of the environment and by areas of skin that would most likely be activated by a physical contact with an object located in that part of the extrapersonal space. This latter feature accounts for the fact that in the superior colliculus the somatosensory representation is primarily skewed towards the nose and face. Thus, the superior colliculus not only codes for saccades, but tends to code specifically for those saccades that are triggered by stimuli of immediate behavioural significance as well as having a more widespread function in orienting responses. This role for the superior colliculus is reflected in its efferent connections to a number of brainstem structures as well as the spinal cord (tectospinal tract). Clinically, damage is rarely confined to this structure but when it is there is a profound loss of saccadic eye movements with neglect.

Lateral geniculate nucleus

The **LGN** consists of six layers in primates, with each layer receiving an input from either the ipsilateral or contralateral eye. The inner two with their large neurones form the magnocellular laminae while the remaining four layers constitute the parvocellular laminae. The morphological distinction between the neurones in these two laminae is also found electrophysiologically.

The parvocellular neurones display chromatic or colour sensitivity and sensitivity to high spatial frequency (detail) with sustained responses to visual stimuli. In contrast, the magnocellular neurones show no colour selectivity, respond best to low spatial frequencies and often have a transient response on being stimulated. Thus, the magnocellular layer neurones have similar properties to the Y ganglion cells and the parvocellular neurones to the X ganglion cells, a similarity that is reflected in the retinogeniculate projection of these two classes of ganglion cells. The X ganglion cells and the parvocellular laminae neurones are responsible for the detection of colour and form (or *P*attern) and constitute the **P channel**, while the **M channel** of the Y ganglion cells and the magnocellular laminae of the LGN are responsible primarily for motion detection (or *M*ovement).

The LGN mainly projects to the **V1** where the afferent fibres synapse in layer IV, and to a lesser extent layer VI, with the M and P channels having different synaptic targets within these laminae. In addition, there is a projection from cells that lie between the laminae of the LGN (intralaminar part of the LGN) direct to layers II and III of V1 (see Chapter 27).

Pretectal structures and the pupillary response to light

There is a projection from the optic tract to the pretectal nuclei of the midbrain which in turn projects bilaterally to the Edinger–Westphal nucleus which provides the parasympathetic input to the pupil allowing it to constrict. Light shone in one eye will cause constriction of both pupils (direct and consensual response). Damage to one of the optic nerves will cause a reduced direct and consensual response but that same eye will constrict normally to light shone in the unaffected eye, producing a ***relative afferent pupillary defect***.

Suprachiasmatic nucleus of the hypothalamus

This nucleus receives a direct retinal input and is important in the generation and control of circadian rhythms (see Chapter 17).

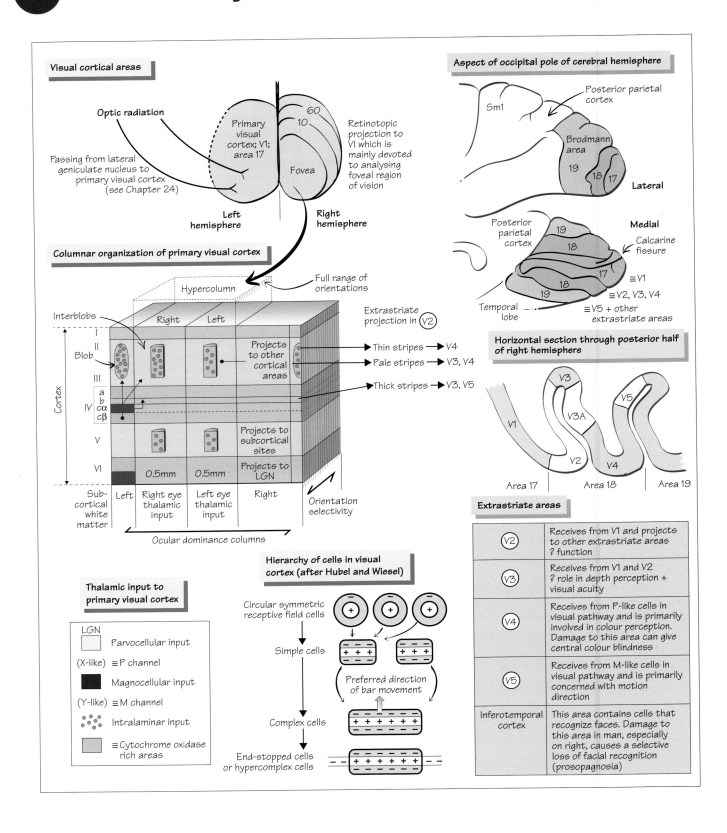

Primary visual cortex (V1 or Brodmann's area 17)

The primary visual cortex (V1) lies along the calcarine fissure of the occipital lobe and receives its major input from the lateral geniculate nucleus (LGN). These connections are organized **retinotopically** so that adjacent areas of the retina project up the visual pathway via neighbouring axons. However, this retinal projection is not a simple map, as the critical factor is the relationship of the photoreceptors to the projecting ganglion cell of the retina. This means that the centre of vision (especially the fovea) dominates the retinal projection to V1 because of the near one-to-one relationship of photoreceptor to ganglion cell at the fovea in contrast to the peripheral retina (see Chapter 25).

The LGN projection to V1 is mainly to layer IV and is different for the M and P channels, while the projection from the intralaminar part of the LGN is to layers II and III of V1 (see below). The LGN input to layer IV of V1 is so great that this cortical layer is futher subdivided into IVa, IVb, IVcα and IVcβ, with each subdivision having slightly different connections. However, in general the cortical neurones in layer IVc of V1 have **centre surround or circular symmetric receptive field organization** (see Chapter 25). These layer IVc neurones then project on to other adjacent neurones within the cortex, in such a way that several neurones of this type converge on to a single neurone whose receptive field is now more complex in terms of the stimulus that best activates it. These cells respond most effectively to a line or bar of illumination of a given orientation and are termed **simple cells**. These cells in turn project in a convergent fashion on to other neurones (**complex cells**), which are predominantly found in layers II and III, and which are maximally activated by stimuli of a given orientation moving in a particular direction, that direction often being orthogonal to the line orientation.

The complex cells project to the **hypercomplex or end-stopped cells** which respond to a line of a given orientation and length. This series of cells originally described by Hubel and Wiesel are thus organized in a hierarchical fashion, with each cell deriving its receptive field from the cells immediately beneath it in the hierarchy.

Hubel and Wiesel further discovered that these neurones were organized into columns of cells with similar properties; the two properties that they originally studied being the eye that provides the dominant input to that neurone (giving **ocular dominance columns**) and the orientation of the line needed to activate neurones maximally (giving **orientation selective columns**). They represented these two sets of columns as running orthogonal to each other, and the area of cortex containing an ocular dominance column from each eye with a complete set of orientation selective columns being termed the **hypercolumn**. This hypercolumn, which is 1 mm² in size, is capable of analysing a given section of the visual field that is defined by the corresponding retinal inputs from both eyes. In the case of the fovea, where there is near unity of photoreceptors to ganglion cells, this visual field is very small, while the converse is true for more peripheral retinal inputs. Therefore a shift of 1 mm in the cortex from one hypercolumn to another leads to a shift in the location of the visual field being analysed, with most of these being concerned with foveal vision (see below).

However, there are two main complicating factors with this model. One is the accommodation of the M and P channels and the second relates to the discovery of cytochrome oxidase (a marker of metabolic activity) -rich areas in layers II, III and IVb (and, to a lesser extent, layers V and VI) which show no orientation selectivity but colour and high spatial frequency sensitivity. These cytochrome oxidase-rich areas in layers II and III are grouped together to form '**blobs**', at least one of which is associated with each ocular dominance column, with the areas between them being termed **interblobs**. Both the blobs and interblobs, together with the cytochrome-rich layer IVb, have distinct projections to V2 and other extrastriate areas—projections that correlate well with the M and P channels. This arrangement of channels and connections suggests that visual information is processed not so much in a hierarchical fashion, but by a series of parallel pathways (see Chapter 15).

The major function of V1, apart from being the first site of binocular interactions, is to deconstruct the visual field into small line segments of various orientation as well as segregating and integrating components of the visual image which can then be relayed to more specialist visual areas. These areas perform more complex visual analysis but rely on their interaction with V1 for the conscious perception of the whole visual image. This occasionally presents itself clinically in patients with bilateral damage to V1, in which they deny being able to see any visual stimulus even though on formal testing they are capable of localizing visual targets accurately (a phenomenon known as *blindsight*).

Visual association or extrastriate areas

The **extrastriate areas** are those cortical areas outside V1 that are primarily involved in visual processing. The number of such areas varies from species to species, with the greatest number being found in humans. These areas are found within Brodmann's areas 18 and 19 and the inferotemporal cortex and are involved in more complex visual processing than V1, with one aspect of the visual scene tending to be dominant in terms of the analysis undertaken by that cortical area (e.g. colour or motion detection). In general, damage to these areas tends to produce complex visual deficits, such as the ability to recognize objects visually (visual agnosia) or selective attributes of the image such as colour (central achromatopsia) or motion. In addition, there are a number of other parts of the CNS that are associated with the visual system including the **posterior parietal cortex** (see Chapter 32); **the frontal cortex and frontal eye fields** (see Chapters 32 and 42); and the subcortical structures of the **hypothalamus** (see Chapter 17) and **upper brainstem** (see Chapter 26).

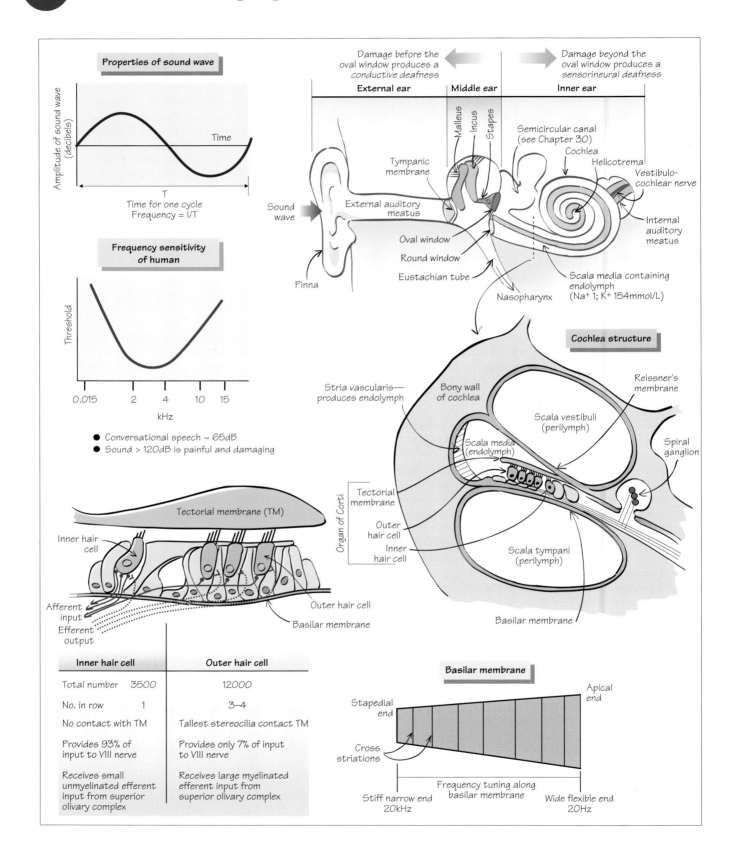

Properties of sound wave

Amplitude of sound wave (decibels) vs Time

T
Time for one cycle
Frequency = I/T

Frequency sensitivity of human

Threshold vs kHz

0.015   2   4   10   15

kHz

- Conversational speech ~ 65dB
- Sound > 120dB is painful and damaging

Damage before the oval window produces a conductive deafness

Damage beyond the oval window produces a sensorineural deafness

| External ear | Middle ear | Inner ear |

Malleus
Incus
Stapes

Semicircular canal (see Chapter 30)
Cochlea
Helicotrema
Vestibulo-cochlear nerve

Tympanic membrane

Sound wave

External auditory meatus

Oval window
Round window
Eustachian tube

Internal auditory meatus

Scala media containing endolymph (Na+ 1; K+ 154mmol/L)

Pinna

Nasopharynx

Cochlea structure

Stria vascularis—produces endolymph

Bony wall of cochlea

Reissner's membrane

Scala vestibuli (perilymph)

Scala media (endolymph)

Spiral ganglion

Organ of Corti

Tectorial membrane

Outer hair cell

Inner hair cell

Scala tympani (perilymph)

Basilar membrane

Tectorial membrane (TM)

Inner hair cell

Afferent input
Efferent output

Outer hair cell
Basilar membrane

	Inner hair cell	Outer hair cell
Total number	3500	12000
No. in row	1	3–4
No contact with TM		Tallest stereocilia contact TM
	Provides 93% of input to VIII nerve	Provides only 7% of input to VIII nerve
	Receives small unmyelinated efferent input from superior olivary complex	Receives large myelinated efferent input from superior olivary complex

Basilar membrane

Stapedial end

Apical end

Cross striations

Frequency tuning along basilar membrane

Stiff narrow end 20kHz

Wide flexible end 20Hz

The **auditory system** is responsible for sound perception. The receptive end-organ is the cochlea of the inner ear which converts sound waves into electrical signals by a process of mechanotransduction. The electrical signal generated in response to a sound is passed (together with information from the vestibular system; see Chapter 30) via the eighth cranial nerve (vestibulocochlear nerve) to the brainstem where it synapses in the cochlear nuclear complex (see Chapter 29).

Although the auditory system as a whole performs many functions, the primary site responsible for frequency discrimination is at the level of the cochlea.

Properties of sound waves

A **sound wave** is characterized by its **amplitude** or **loudness** (measured in decibels [dB]), **frequency** or **pitch** (measured in hertz [Hz]), **waveform**, **phase** and **quality** or **timbre**. The intensity of sound can vary enormously but in general we can discriminate changes in intensity of around 1–2 dB.

The arrival of a sound at the head creates phase and intensity differences between the two ears unless the sound originates from the midline. The degree of delay and intensity change between the two ears as a result of their physical separation is useful but probably not necessary for the localization of sounds (see Chapter 29).

External and middle ear

On reaching the ear the sound passes down the **external auditory meatus** to the **tympanic membrane or eardrum**, which vibrates at a frequency and strength determined by the impinging sound. This causes the **three ear ossicles** in the **middle ear** to move, displacing fluid within the **cochlea** as the stapedial foot process moves within the oval window of the cochlea. This process is essential in reducing the acoustic impedance of the system and in enhancing the response to sound, because a sound hitting a fluid directly is largely reflected.

There are two small muscles associated with the ear ossicles, which protect them from damage by loud noises as well as modifying the movement of the stapedial foot process in the oval window. Damage to the ear ossicles (e.g. *otosclerosis*), middle ear (e.g. infection or *otitis media*) or external auditory meatus (e.g. blockage by wax) all lead to a reduction in hearing or *deafness* that is **conductive** in nature.

Inner ear and cochlea

The displacement of the stapedial foot process in the **oval window** generates waves in the perilymph-filled scala vestibuli and tympani of the cochlea. These two scalae are in communication at the apical end of the cochlea, the helicotrema, but are separated for the rest of their length by the scala media which contains the transduction apparatus in the organ of Corti.

The organ of Corti sits on the floor of the scala media on a structure known as the **basilar membrane (BM)**, the width of which increases with distance from the stapedial end. This increase in width coupled to a decrease in stiffness of the BM means that sounds of high frequency maximally displace the BM at the stapedial end of the cochlea while low-frequency sounds maximally activate the apical end of the BM. Thus, frequency tuning is, in part, a function of the BM although it is greatly enhanced and made more selective by the hair cells of the organ of Corti that lie on this membrane.

The **organ of Corti** is a complex structure that contains the cells of **auditory transduction**, the **hair cells** (see Chapter 21), which are of two types in this structure: a single row of **inner hair cells** (IHCs) which provide most of the signal in the eighth cranial nerve; and 3–4 rows of **outer hair cells** (OHCs) which have a role in modulating the response of IHCs to a given sound. These two types of hair cells are morphologically and electrophysiologically distinct. While the IHCs receive little input from the brainstem, the OHCs do so in the form of an input from the superior olivary complex which has the effect of modifying the shape and response properties of these cells. Some of the OHCs make direct contact with the overlying **tectorial membrane (TM)** in the organ of Corti which may be important in modifying the response of the IHCs to sound, as these cells do not contact the TM but do provide 93% of the afferent input of the cochlear nerve. One afferent fibre receives from many OHCs, but a single IHC is associated with many afferent fibres. In addition to these differences between OHCs and IHCs, there are subtle alterations in the hair cells themselves with distance along the scala media. These alterations in shape alter their tuning characteristics which adds a degree of refinement to frequency tuning beyond that imparted by the resonance properties of the BM.

Damage to the cochlea, hair cells or cochlear part of the vestibulocochlear nerve leads to *deafness* that is described as being **sensorineural** in nature. Trauma, ischaemia and tumours of the eighth cranial nerve can all cause this. Certain hereditary causes of deafness have been associated recently with defects in the proteins found in the stereocilia of hair cells (see also Chapter 21).

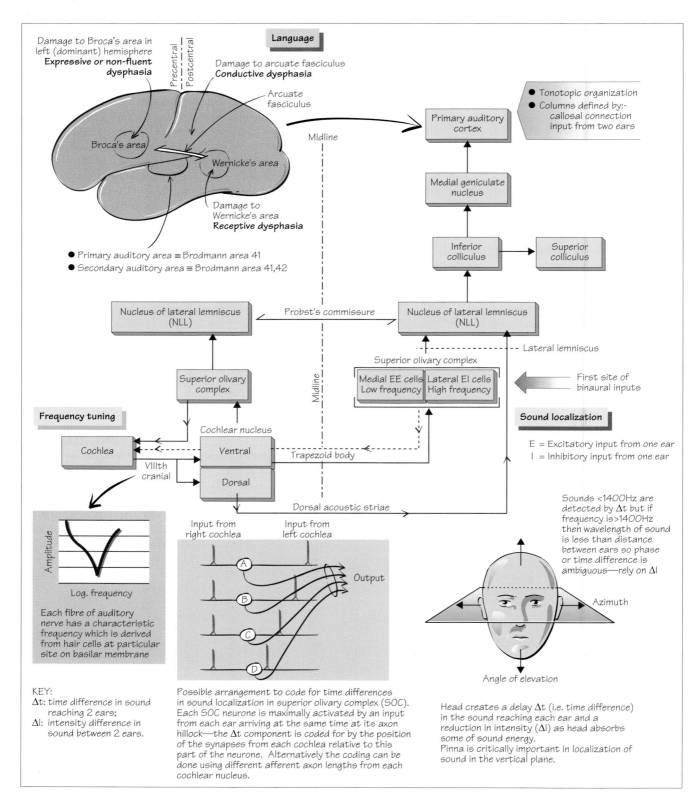

Language

Damage to Broca's area in left (dominant) hemisphere **Expressive or non-fluent dysphasia**

Precentral Postcentral

Damage to arcuate fasciculus **Conductive dysphasia**

Arcuate fasciculus

Broca's area

Wernicke's area

Midline

Damage to Wernicke's area **Receptive dysphasia**

● Primary auditory area ≡ Brodmann area 41
● Secondary auditory area ≡ Brodmann area 41,42

● Tonotopic organization
● Columns defined by:- callosal connection input from two ears

Primary auditory cortex

Medial geniculate nucleus

Inferior colliculus → Superior colliculus

Nucleus of lateral lemniscus (NLL) — Probst's commissure — Nucleus of lateral lemniscus (NLL)

Lateral lemniscus

Superior olivary complex

Medial EE cells Low frequency | Lateral EI cells High frequency

First site of binaural inputs

Midline

Frequency tuning

Sound localization

Cochlear nucleus

Cochlea — Ventral

VIIIth cranial — Trapezoid body

Dorsal

E = Excitatory input from one ear
I = Inhibitory input from one ear

Dorsal acoustic striae

Amplitude / Log. frequency

Each fibre of auditory nerve has a characteristic frequency which is derived from hair cells at particular site on basilar membrane

Input from right cochlea | Input from left cochlea

A
B
C
D

Output

Sounds <1400Hz are detected by Δt but if frequency is >1400Hz then wavelength of sound is less than distance between ears so phase or time difference is ambiguous—rely on ΔI

Azimuth

Angle of elevation

KEY:
Δt: time difference in sound reaching 2 ears;
ΔI: intensity difference in sound between 2 ears.

Possible arrangement to code for time differences in sound localization in superior olivary complex (SOC). Each SOC neurone is maximally activated by an input from each ear arriving at the same time at its axon hillock—the Δt component is coded for by the position of the synapses from each cochlea relative to this part of the neurone. Alternatively the coding can be done using different afferent axon lengths from each cochlear nucleus.

Head creates a delay Δt (i.e. time difference) in the sound reaching each ear and a reduction in intensity (ΔI) as head absorbs some of sound energy.
Pinna is critically important in localization of sound in the vertical plane.

The **vestibulocochlear or eighth cranial nerve** transmits information from both the cochlea and vestibular apparatus; the latter is discussed in Chapter 30. Each fibre of the cochlear nerve is selectively tuned to a characteristic frequency, which is determined by its site of origin within the cochlea (see Chapter 28). These fibres are then arranged according to the location of their innervating hair cells along the basilar membrane (BM), and this tonotopic organization is maintained throughout the auditory pathway.

On entering the brainstem the cochlear nerve synapses in the cochlear nuclear complex of the medulla.

Auditory pathways

The **cochlear nucleus** is divided into a **ventral (VCN)** and **dorsal (DCN)** part. The VCN projects to the **superior olivary complex (SOC)** bilaterally while the DCN projects via the dorsal acoustic striae to the contralateral **nucleus of the lateral lemniscus** and **inferior colliculus**.

The **SOC** contains spindle-shaped neurones with a lateral and medial dendrite, which receive an input from each ear. It is the first site of binaural interactions and so this structure is important in sound localization. In the **medial part of the SOC** this input is excitatory from each ear (**EE cells**) whereas in the **lateral SOC** the neurones have an excitatory input from one ear and an inhibitory input from the other (**EI cells**).

The EE cells by virtue of their input are important in the localization of sounds of low frequency (less than 1.4 kHz) where the critical factor is the delay (Δt) in the sound reaching one and then the other ear. One possible arrangement that could be employed is shown in the figure and relies on the differential localization of the synaptic inputs to a single SOC neurone from the two ears.

The EI cells are important in the localization of higher frequency sounds where the difference in intensity (ΔI) of sound between the two ears is important (ΔI being generated as a result of the head acting as a shield). Sounds of frequencies greater than 1.4 kHz (in the case of humans) rely on ΔI for localization. In the case of sounds originating in the midline, there will be no Δt and no ΔI, and there is some confusion in localization which can be overcome to some extent by moving the head or using other sensory cues.

The localization of sound within the vertical plane is dependent in some way on the pinna.

The SOC not only projects rostrally to the **inferior colliculus (IC)**, but also has an important input to the cochlea where it primarily controls the OHCs and by so doing the response properties of the organ of Corti (see Chapter 28). The projection to the IC is tonotopic and this structure also receives an input from the **primary auditory cortex (A1)** and other sensory modalities. In this respect it interacts with the superior colliculus and is involved in the orienting response to novel audiovisual stimuli (see Chapters 26 and 42).

The IC projects to the **medial geniculate nucleus of the thalamus (MGN)**, which projects to the **A1** in the superior temporal gyrus. This area corresponds to Brodmann's areas 41 and 42, with the thalamic afferent input synapsing in layers III and IV of the cortex. The columnar organization of A1 is poorly defined but the tonotopic map is maintained so that low-frequency sounds are located posteriorly and high-frequency sounds anteriorly.

Secondary auditory cortical areas and language

In A1, apart from neurones with relatively simple afferent inputs, there are some cells that respond to complex sounds. In addition, this area of cortex appears to be activated when one imagines sound and may be the site of auditory hallucinations in patients with schizophrenia (see Chapter 55). The neurones with more complex response properties are more frequently found in the **secondary auditory areas**, where music for example is processed. However, they reach their most complex in humans in **Wernicke's area**, the cortical site of language comprehension. This area is found in the dominant hemisphere (usually left) and when damaged (e.g. in cerebrovascular accidents [CVAs]; see Chapter 19) leads to a *receptive* or *fluent dysphasia*, or an inability to understand what is being said. This area is connected, via the **arcuate fasciculus**, to an area in the dominant hemisphere frontal lobe known as **Broca's area**. This frontal area is responsible for the expression of speech and damage to it causes an *expressive* or *non-fluent dysphasia* which is an inability to speak fluently in the absence of damage to the motor apparatus of articulation. *Aphasia* is an inability to generate any speech and in a large middle cerebral artery CVA of the dominant hemisphere this can occur as both Wernicke's and Broca's areas are involved. Selective lesions of the arcuate fasciculus are said to produce a *conduction aphasia*, where the patient understands and can speak but cannot repeat words and sentences. However, current evidence points to a more complex interaction among brain regions in the recognition and production of speech.

Aphasia and dysphasia are to be distinguished from deficits in the activation and execution of the motor acts of speaking (e.g. weakness of the palate and tongue in *motorneurone disease*), which is termed *dysarthria* (or anarthria when no speech can be generated).

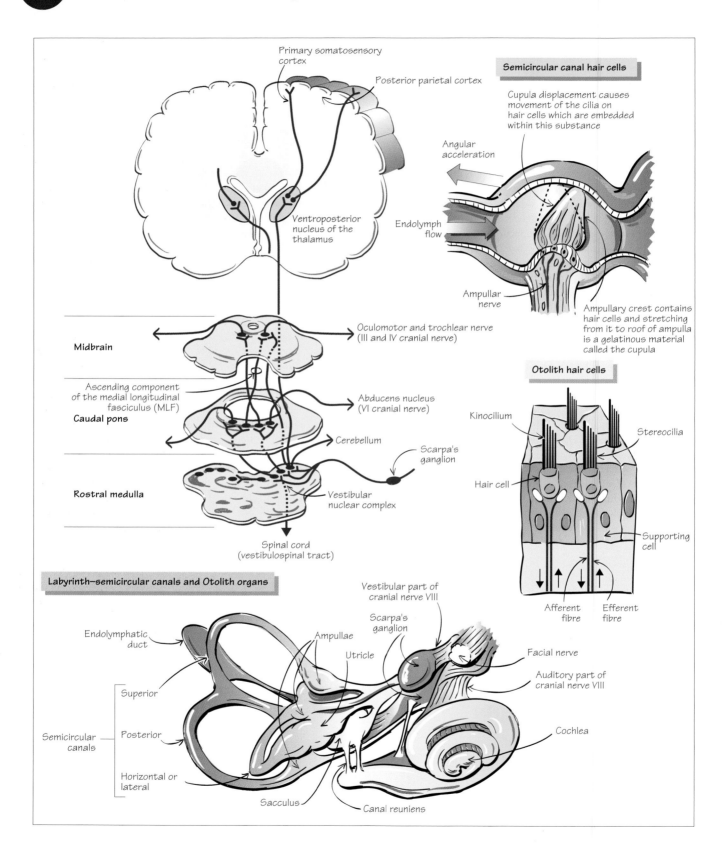

Primary somatosensory cortex

Posterior parietal cortex

Ventroposterior nucleus of the thalamus

Semicircular canal hair cells

Cupula displacement causes movement of the cilia on hair cells which are embedded within this substance

Angular acceleration

Endolymph flow

Ampullar nerve

Ampullary crest contains hair cells and stretching from it to roof of ampulla is a gelatinous material called the cupula

Midbrain

Oculomotor and trochlear nerve (III and IV cranial nerve)

Ascending component of the medial longitudinal fasciculus (MLF)

Caudal pons

Abducens nucleus (VI cranial nerve)

Cerebellum

Scarpa's ganglion

Rostral medulla

Vestibular nuclear complex

Spinal cord (vestibulospinal tract)

Otolith hair cells

Kinocilium

Stereocilia

Hair cell

Supporting cell

Afferent fibre

Efferent fibre

Labyrinth–semicircular canals and Otolith organs

Endolymphatic duct

Ampullae

Scarpa's ganglion

Vestibular part of cranial nerve VIII

Utricle

Facial nerve

Superior

Auditory part of cranial nerve VIII

Semicircular canals

Posterior

Cochlea

Horizontal or lateral

Sacculus

Canal reuniens

The vestibular system is concerned with balance, postural reflexes and eye movements and is one of the oldest systems of the brain. It consists of a peripheral transducer component which projects to the brainstem (including the oculomotor nuclei), and from there to the thalamus and sensory cortex as well as to the cerebellum and spinal cord. Disruption to the system (e.g., *vestibular neuronitis/labyrinthitis*) results in the symptoms of dizziness, vertigo, nausea ± blurred vision with signs of eye movement abnormalities (typically nystagmus; see Chapter 42) and unsteadiness. In the comatose patient, clinical testing of the vestibular system can provide useful information on the integrity of the brainstem as it is associated with a number of primitive brainstem reflexes (see Chapter 13).

Vestibular transduction

The peripheral transducer component consists of the **labyrinth**, which is made up of two **otolith organs** (the **utricle** and the **sacculus**) together with the **ampullae** located in the three **semicircular canals**. The otolith organs are primarily concerned with static head position and linear acceleration while the semicircular canals are more concerned with rotational (angular) acceleration of the head.

Hair cells are found in both the otolith organs and the ampullae and are similar in structure to those found in the cochlea (see Chapters 21 and 28). As in the cochlea, deflection of the **stereocilia** towards the kinocilium depolarizes the cell and allows transmitter to be released from the hair cell, leading to activation of the associated afferent fibre. The converse is true if the stereocilia are deflected in the opposite direction. Movement of the cilia is associated with rotational movement of the head (ampullae receptors in the semicircular canals) and acceleration or tilting of the head (otolith organs in utricle), as although head movement causes the **endolymph** bathing the hair cells to move, it 'lags behind' and so distorts the stereocilia.

Spontaneous activity in the afferent fibres is high, reflecting the spontaneous leakage of transmitter from the cell at the synapse. Hyperpolarization of the hair cell therefore results in a reduced afferent discharge, while depolarization is associated with an increase in firing. Efferent fibres from the brainstem terminating on the hair cells can change the sensitivity of the receptor end-organ.

Peripheral disorders of the vestibular system

Damage to the peripheral vestibular system is not uncommon. An example of such a disorder is *benign positional vertigo* which commonly occurs after trauma or infection of the vestibular apparatus with the deposition of debris (e.g. otolith crystals or otoconia) typically in the posterior semicircular canal. This condition, which is characterized by paroxysms of vertigo, nausea and ataxia induced by turning the head into certain positions—such as lying down or rolling over in bed—is therefore the consequence of distortion of endolymph flow in this canal secondary to the debris. Treatment and cure can be effected if a series of head manoeuvres are followed which allows the debris to fall out of the semicircular canal and into the ampullae. Viral infections of the vestibular apparatus are common (**labyrinthitis**) and can be severely disabling with profound dizziness and vomiting without any head movement. Such infections are usually self-limiting.

Bilateral failure of the vestibular apparatus can result in *oscillopsia*, a symptom describing an inability to visually fixate on objects especially with head movements (see Chapter 42). In contrast, powerful excitation of the vestibular system such as that encountered during motion sickness produces dizziness, vomiting, sweating and tachycardia, caused by discrepancies between vestibular and visual information.

Vestibular function can be tested by introducing water into the external meatus (**caloric testing**). When warm water is applied to a seated subject whose head is tilted back by about 60°, nystagmus towards the treated side is observed. Cold water produces nystagmus towards the opposite side. These effects reflect the changes in the temperature of the endolymph and an effect resembling head rotation away from the irrigated side.

Central vestibular system and vestibular reflexes

Afferent vestibular fibres in the eighth cranial nerve have their cell bodies in the vestibular (**Scarpa's) ganglion** and terminate in one of the **four vestibular nuclei** in the medulla which also receive inputs from neck muscle receptors and the visual system.

The vestibular nuclei project to the spinal cord (see Chapters 12, 34 and 36), contralateral vestibular nuclei, the cerebellum and oculomotor nuclei, and the ipsi- and contralateral thalamus. Some of these structures are important in reflex eye movements such as the ability to maintain visual fixation while moving the head—the vestibulo-ocular reflex (VOR; see Chapters 39, 42 and 50). Other projections of the vestibular nuclei are important in maintaining posture and gait. The cortical termination of the vestibular input to the central nervous system (CNS) is the **primary somatosensory cortex (SmI)** and the **posterior parietal cortex** (see Chapter 32). Very rarely, *epileptic* seizures originating in this area can arise and give symptoms of vestibular disturbance.

Caloric testing of the vestibular system examines the integrity of the vestibular apparatus and its brainstem connections so it can be useful in comatosed patients when the degree of brainstem function needs to be ascertained. Less severe central damage to the vestibular apparatus can occur in a number of conditions including *multiple sclerosis* (see Chapter 59) and vascular insults (see Chapter 19). In most cases other structures are involved and so there are other symptoms and signs on examination.

31 Olfaction and taste

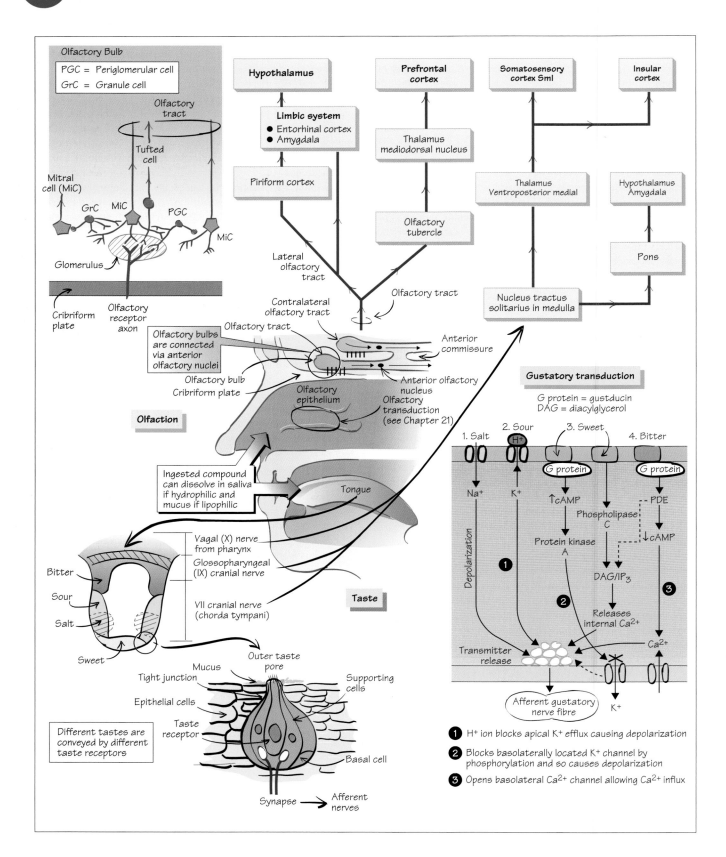

Olfactory Bulb

PGC = Periglomerular cell
GrC = Granule cell

Olfactory tract

Tufted cell

Mitral cell (MiC)

GrC MiC PGC MiC

Glomerulus

Cribriform plate

Olfactory receptor axon

Hypothalamus

Limbic system
- Entorhinal cortex
- Amygdala

Piriform cortex

Prefrontal cortex

Thalamus mediodorsal nucleus

Olfactory tubercle

Somatosensory cortex SmI

Thalamus Ventroposterior medial

Insular cortex

Hypothalamus Amygdala

Pons

Nucleus tractus solitarius in medulla

Lateral olfactory tract

Contralateral olfactory tract

Olfactory tract

Olfactory bulbs are connected via anterior olfactory nuclei

Olfactory tract

Anterior commissure

Olfactory bulb

Cribriform plate

Anterior olfactory nucleus

Olfactory epithelium

Olfactory transduction (see Chapter 21)

Olfaction

Gustatory transduction

G protein = gustducin
DAG = diacylglycerol

1. Salt   2. Sour   3. Sweet   4. Bitter

G protein   G protein

Na⁺   K⁺   ↑cAMP   Phospholipase C   PDE

Depolarization

Protein kinase A   ↓cAMP

1   **2**   DAG/IP₃

Releases internal Ca²⁺

Ca²⁺

Transmitter release

Afferent gustatory nerve fibre

K⁺

Ingested compound can dissolve in saliva if hydrophilic and mucus if lipophilic

Tongue

Vagal (X) nerve from pharynx

Glossopharyngeal (IX) cranial nerve

VII cranial nerve (chorda tympani)

Bitter

Sour

Salt

Sweet

Taste

Outer taste pore

Mucus

Tight junction

Epithelial cells

Taste receptor

Different tastes are conveyed by different taste receptors

Supporting cells

Basal cell

Synapse → Afferent nerves

1 H⁺ ion blocks apical K⁺ efflux causing depolarization

2 Blocks basolaterally located K⁺ channel by phosphorylation and so causes depolarization

3 Opens basolateral Ca²⁺ channel allowing Ca²⁺ influx

The **olfactory or first cranial nerve** contains more fibres than any other sensory nerve projecting to the central nervous system (CNS), while **taste** is relayed via the seventh, ninth and tenth cranial nerves (see Chapter 14).

Olfaction

The olfactory system as a whole is able to discriminate a great diversity of different chemical stimuli or odours, and this is made possible through thousands of different **olfactory receptors**. These receptors are located in the apical dendrite of the olfactory receptor cell and the axon of this cell projects directly into the CNS via the **cribriform plate** at the top of the nose to the olfactory bulb.

The **olfactory stimulus or odour**, on binding to the olfactory receptor, depolarizes it (see Chapter 21) which, if sufficient, leads to the generation of action potentials at the cell body which are then conducted down the olfactory nerve axons to the olfactory bulb.

The **olfactory nerve** passes through the roof of the nose through a bone known as the cribriform plate. Damage to this structure (e.g. head trauma) can shear the olfactory nerve axons causing a loss of smell or *anosmia*. However, the most common cause of a loss of smell is local trouble within the nose, usually infection and inflammation. The olfactory receptor axons then synapse in the olfactory bulb that lies at the base of the frontal lobe. Damage to this structure, as occurs in frontal *meningiomas*, produces anosmia that can be unilateral.

The **olfactory bulb** contains a complex arrangement of cells. The axons from the olfactory nerve synapse on the apical dendrites of mitral and, to a lesser extent, tufted cells, both of which project out of the olfactory bulb as the olfactory tract. The olfactory bulb contains a number of inhibitory interneurones (granule and periglomerular cells) which are important in modifying the flow of olfactory information through the bulb. Some of these neurones are replaced throughout life, with the neural precursor cells for them originating in the subventricular zone and then migrating to the olfactory bulb via the rostral migratory stream, a structure that definitely exists in some adult mammalian brains including humans. This system may be important in olfactory learning.

The **olfactory tract** projects to the temporal lobe where it synapses in the **pyriform cortex** and **limbic system**, which projects to the **hypothalamus**. This projection is important in the behavioural effects of olfaction, which are perhaps more evident in other species. In humans, lesions in these structures rarely produce a pure anosmia, but activation of this area of the CNS as occurs in *temporal lobe epilepsy* (see Chapter 58) is associated with the abnormal perception of smells (e.g. olfactory hallucinations).

The projection of the olfactory system to the thalamus is small and is via the olfactory tubercle to the mediodorsal nucleus, which projects to the prefrontal cortex. The role of this pathway is not clear.

Taste

The **taste** or **gustatory receptors** are located in the tongue. They are clustered together in fungiform papillae with support and stem cells; the latter dividing to replace those gustatory receptors that are damaged. The apical surface of the gustatory receptor contains microvilli covered in mucus, which is generated by the neighbouring goblet cells. Any ingested compound can therefore reach the gustatory receptor; hydrophilic substances are dissolved in saliva while lipophilic substances are dissolved in the mucus. Taste is traditionally classified according to four modalities—salt, sour, sweet and bitter—which correlate well with the different transduction processes that are now known to exist for these different tastes. A fifth taste (umami) has also recently been described.

Salt stimuli cause a direct depolarization of the gustatory receptors by virtue of the fact that Na^+ passes through an amiloride-sensitive apical membrane channel. The depolarization leads to the release of neurotransmitter from the basal part of the cell which activates the afferent fibres in the relevant cranial nerve. **Sour stimuli**, in contrast, probably achieve a similar effect by the blocking of apical voltage-dependent H^+ channels. **Sweet stimuli** bind to a receptor that activates the G protein, gustducin, which then activates an adenylate cyclase with cyclic adenosine monophosphate (cAMP) production. The rise in cAMP activates a protein kinase that phosphorylates and closes basolateral K^+ channels and by so doing depolarizes the receptor. **Bitter stimuli** similarly rely on receptor binding and G-protein activation. One pathway involves gustducin but, in this instance, this leads to activation of a cAMP phosphodiesterase that reduces the level of cAMP (and so the phosphorylating protein kinase) leading to opening of the basolateral Ca^{2+} channels and so transmitter release. An alternative pathway for both sweet and bitter tastes involves the activation of a phospholipase C and the production of inositol triphosphate (IP_3) and diacylglycerol (DAG) which can release Ca^{2+} from internal stores within the receptor. The increased Ca^{2+} concentration promotes neurotransmitter release.

The receptors relay their information via the **chorda tympani** (anterior two-thirds of the tongue) and **glossopharyngeal nerve** (posterior third of the tongue) to **the nucleus of the solitary tract** in the medulla (see Chapters 13 and 14). The structure projects rostrally via the thalamus to the primary somatosensory cortex (SmI) and the insular cortex, with a possible further projection to the hypothalamus and amygdala. Some patients with *temporal lobe epilepsy* have an aura of an abnormal taste in the mouth which may relate to abnormal electrical activity within the temporal lobe (see Chapter 58).

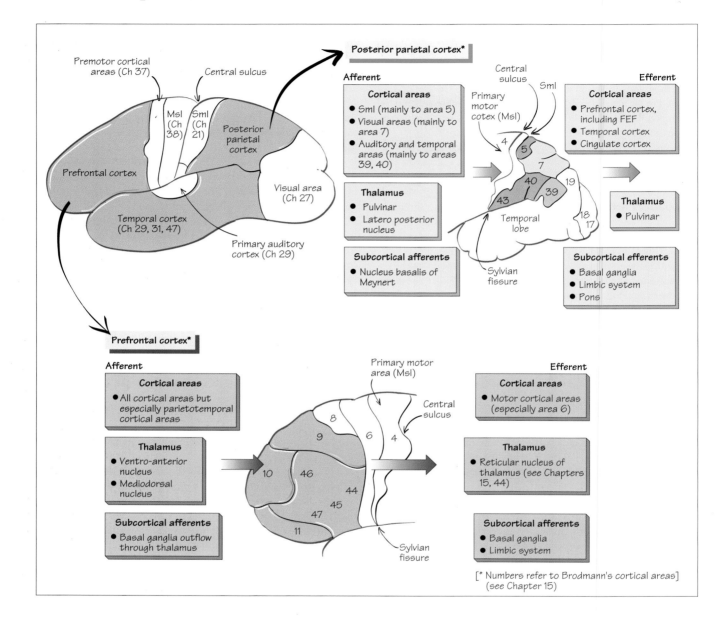

The **association cortices** are those parts of the cerebral cortex that do not have a primary motor or sensory role, but instead are involved in the higher order processing of sensory information necessary for perception and movement initiation.

These association areas include the posterior parietal cortex (PPC; defined in monkeys as corresponding to Brodmann's areas 5 and 7, and in humans including areas 39 and 40); the prefrontal cortex (corresponding to Brodmann's areas 9–12 and 44–47); and the temporal cortex (corresponding to Brodmann's areas 21, 22, 37 and 41–43). The temporal cortex is involved in audition and language, complex visual processing (such as face recognition) and memory and is discussed in Chapters 27, 29, 46 and 47.

Posterior parietal cortex

This area has developed greatly during evolution and is related to specific forms of human behaviour, such as the extensive use of tools, collaborative strategic planning and the development of language. It has two main subdivisions within it: one involved mainly with somatosensory information (centred on area 5); and the other with visual stimuli (centred on area 7).

Neurophysiologically, **area 5** contains many units with a complex sensory input often with a convergence of different sensory modalities, such as proprioceptive and cutaneous stimuli. These units with such a dual input are probably involved in the sensory control of posture and movements. Other units with multiple cutaneous inputs are probably

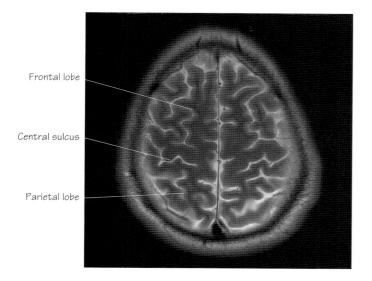

Frontal lobe

Central sulcus

Parietal lobe

more involved in object recognition. However, in addition to having these complex sensory inputs, units in this area are often only maximally activated when the sensory stimulus is of interest or behavioural significance. Damage to this area produces a contralateral sensory loss that is often subtle, e.g. a failure to recognize objects on tactile manipulation (*astereognosis*). In addition, patients often demonstrate an **inattention** to stimuli received on the contralateral side of the body. This can be so severe that the patient denies the existence of that part of his or her body which can then interfere with the actions of the normal non-neglected side (intermanual conflict or alien limb). More commonly, the patient fails to perceive sensory stimuli contralaterally when stimuli are simultaneously applied to both sides of the body (extinction).

In contrast, **area 7** is more involved in complex visual processing, with many of the units in this area responding to stimuli of interest or behavioural significance (e.g. food). Many different units are found in this cortical area some of which maximally respond to the visual fixation and tracking, while others are more involved in the process of switching attention from one visual object of interest to another (light sensitive or visual space neurones). There are individual neurones in area 7 that respond to both sensory and visual stimuli. Some of these neurones are maximally activated when a stimulus is moved towards the neurone's cutaneous receptive field from extrapersonal (distant) space, while others are maximally activated during visual fixation of a desired object in which there is concomitant movement of the arm towards that object. In humans, damage to this area produces a neglect of visual stimuli in the contralateral hemifield, as well as defects in eye movement and the visual control of movement. However, a more striking deficit that may occur in some patients is in the realm of complex visual processing such as route finding, the construction of complex

shapes and the copying of genesis of motor actions/gestures (*dyspraxia*).

Finally, in humans, and to a lesser extent in other primates and animals, units are found in the PPC that are maximally activated by vestibular and auditory inputs (see Chapters 29 and 30). Therefore damage to this area in humans can lead to complex difficulties in vision and visually guided movements, balance and language processing, including arithmetic skills. This includes an inability to write (*agraphia*), to read (*alexia*) and calculate simple sums (*acalculia*).

Prefrontal cortex

This cortical area has increased in size with phylogenetic development and has its greatest representation in humans. It is involved in the purposive behaviour of an organism and thus is intimately involved in the planning of responses to stimuli that include a motor component (see Chapter 34). Within this structure are specialized cortical areas such as the frontal eye fields (FEF; see Chapter 42) and Broca's area (see Chapter 29). Although the prefrontal cortex is treated as a functional whole, this is a gross simplification.

Many different types of units are encountered neurophysiologically in this area of cortex, but they generally respond to complex sensory stimuli of behaviourial relevance, which can then be translated into a cue for movement.

Damage to this site in animals leads to increased distractability with corresponding deficits in working memory (the ability to retain information for more than a few seconds) and a change in locomotor activity and emotional responsiveness. A patient with frontal lobe damage anterior to the motor areas has a characteristic syndrome without insight (as occurs in frontal variant **Fronto Temporal Dementia** (FTD)). The patient is often disinhibited, which results in him or her behaving in an atypical, often childish, fashion. The patient has very poor attention and is easily distractable, cannot retain information and is sometimes unable to form new memories, with a tendency to perseverate (the repetition of words or phrases and actions) and pursue old patterns of behaviour even in the face of environmental change. He or she is unable to formulate and pursue goals and plans, to generalize and deduce, and may have difficulties in judging risk. There is often a marked reduction in verbal output, which is also reflected in motor behaviour as evidenced by a lack of spontaneous movement with a change in food preference, typically favouring sweet over savoury foods. The patient can become apathetic with severe blunting of his or her emotional responses, although in some cases the converse is true with the patient becoming aggressive. Overall, the patient's personality changes and it is typically others who bring the patient to medical attention, as the patient usually denies there is any problem (no insight).

The reliance on the clinical symptomatology to describe the function of the prefrontal cortex relates to the fact that this part of the cortex is most developed in humans. However, extensive damage of the frontal lobes can also affect the cortical motor areas (see Chapter 37), eye movements (see Chapter 42), the ability to talk (an expressive dysphasia; see Chapter 29) and the control of micturition.

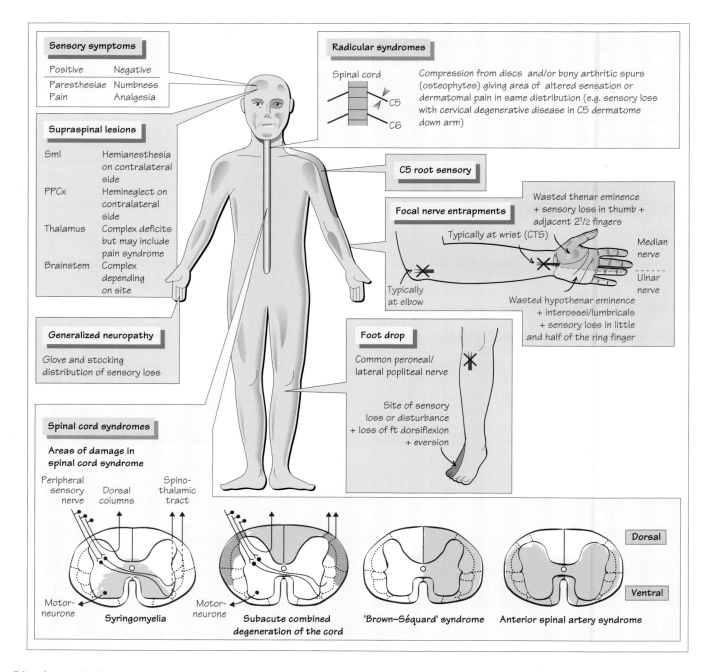

Sensory symptoms

Positive	Negative
Paresthesiae	Numbness
Pain	Analgesia

Supraspinal lesions

Sml	Hemianesthesia on contralateral side
PPCx	Hemineglect on contralateral side
Thalamus	Complex deficits but may include pain syndrome
Brainstem	Complex depending on site

Generalized neuropathy

Glove and stocking distribution of sensory loss

Spinal cord syndromes

Areas of damage in spinal cord syndrome

Peripheral sensory nerve Dorsal columns Spino-thalamic tract

Motor-neurone Syringomyelia

Motor-neurone Subacute combined degeneration of the cord

'Brown–Séquard' syndrome

Anterior spinal artery syndrome

Dorsal

Ventral

Radicular syndromes

Spinal cord

C5
C6

Compression from discs and/or bony arthritic spurs (osteophytes) giving area of altered sensation or dermatomal pain in same distribution (e.g. sensory loss with cervical degenerative disease in C5 dermatome down arm)

C5 root sensory

Focal nerve entrapments

Typically at wrist (CTS)

Typically at elbow

Wasted thenar eminence + sensory loss in thumb + adjacent 2½ fingers

Median nerve

Ulnar nerve

Wasted hypothenar eminence + interossei/lumbricals + sensory loss in little and half of the ring finger

Foot drop

Common peroneal/ lateral popliteal nerve

Site of sensory loss or disturbance + loss of ft dorsiflexion + eversion

Disturbances in the sensory pathways can produce one of two main symptoms: negative ones, with a loss of sensation such as numbness or analgesia; or positive ones, such as pins and needles (paresthesiae) or pain. These symptoms can arise from many different sites along the sensory pathways, but it is often the distribution of sensory change that points towards the likely site of pathology.

In order to determine the nature and cause of the sensory disturbance a full history and examination is needed along with appropriate tests. Most patients with isolated sensory symptoms do not yield to a diagnosis but the most common causes are neuropathies and multiple sclerosis.

A typical screen of tests for patients with sensory symptoms involves blood tests, nerve conduction studies (NCS) and magnetic resonance imaging (MRI) of brain and spinal cord. In all cases it is important to remember that non-neurological causes, e.g. hyperventilation, will give positive sensory symptoms, typically in the fingers and peri-orally.

Peripheral nerve

Diseases of the peripheral nerves can cause sensory disturbance. This can either be caused by *focal nerve entrapment* or a *generalized neuropathy*, in which case the disease process can target either the large or small fibres or both.

Common focal nerve entrapments include:
- The median nerve at the wrist (*carpel tunnel syndrome*). Patients typically present with aching in the forearm especially at night, weakness of some of the thumb muscles (so causing problems with such things as taking lids off jars) and loss of sensation over the thumb and adjacent two and a half fingers. It often resolves spontaneously but in cases where it does not, simple splinting, steroid injection or even surgical decompression is often curative.
- The ulnar nerve at the elbow. Patients present with wasting of most of the intrinsic hand muscles with weakness and loss of sensation in the hand involving the little and half of the ring finger but without involvement of the forearm. It can be treated by surgical transposition of the nerve in some cases.
- The common peroneal (or lateral popliteal nerve) can be trapped around the knee. Patients typically present with foot drop and numbness on the outer aspect of the foot.

Generalized neuropathies may be caused by many disorders and if large fibres are preferentially involved then there is a loss of joint position sense, vibration perception and light touch along with absent or reduced reflexes. These neuropathies are rarely purely sensory in nature so are often associated with weakness and wasting. The typical pattern of sensory loss in these neuropathies is 'glove and stocking' which, as the name implies, reflects the symmetrical loss of sensation in all four limbs to the forearm and to the ankle or shin.

In some cases patients complain of much pain but paradoxically have reduced sensation for pain and temperature. These patients are more likely to have a *small fibre neuropathy*.

Rarely, the dorsal root ganglion cell (as opposed to the peripheral nerve) is targeted by the disease process. In these instances there is a devastating loss of proprioception which greatly compromises motor function.

Peripheral pain syndromes are discussed in Chapters 23 and 24, but it is always important to remember that pain is more often the result of non-neurological causes such as arthritis or local tissue damage.

The nerves as they emerge out of the spinal column can be trapped typically by bony spurs or intravertebral discs and give sensory disturbance along that nerve root. Patients normally complain of pain radiating down that nerve root with sensory abnormalities confined to that dermatome (see Chapter 1). This commonly happens in the cervical and lumbar region and may require surgical decompression especially in cases where there is weakness, wasting and loss of the appropriate reflexes caused by compression of the merging spinal nerve root.

Spinal cord

The different courses of the spinal pathways for sensation can lead to distinctive syndromes.

Syringomyelia

Syringomyelia is the development, for a number of reasons, of a cyst or cavity around or near to the central canal, usually in the cervical region, which tends to spread over time up and down the spinal cord. The lesion typically disrupts the spinothalamic tract (STT) fibres as they cross just ventral to the central canal, resulting in a dissociated sensory loss, i.e. reduced temperature and pain sensation at the level of the lesion but normal light touch, vibration perception and joint position sense (see Chapter 22). In addition, there may be motor involvement because of expansion of the cyst into the ventral horn or dorsolaterally into the descending motor tracts and other ascending sensory pathways.

Subacute combined degeneration of the spinal cord

This is usually associated with pernicious anaemia and a lack of vitamin B_{12}. It is characterized by demyelination and eventually degeneration of the dorsal columns (DCs), the spinocerebellar tracts and the corticospinal tract (CoST) and in addition there is damage to peripheral nerves (*peripheral neuropathy*). Patients therefore develop a combination of paraesthesiae and sensory loss (especially light touch, vibration perception and joint position sense) with weakness and incoordination (see Chapter 22). The weakness may be of both an upper *and* lower motor neurone type (see Chapters 34 and 43).

Brown–Séquard syndrome

This describes a lesion involving half of the cord such that there is an ipsilateral loss of position and tactile senses (DC sensory information), a contralateral loss of temperature sensation originating from several segments below the lesion (STT sensory information), and ipsilateral spasticity and weakness because of involvement of the CoST pathway (see Chapters 22 and 23).

Anterior spinal artery syndrome

This syndrome describes the situation when there is occlusion of the artery providing blood to the anterior two-thirds of the cord. The patient has weakness and sensory loss to temperature and pain with preservation of DC sensory modalities such as joint position sense and vibration perception (see Chapter 19).

Transverse myelitis

Transverse myelitis (not shown in figure) describes a complete lesion of the whole spinal cord at one level that produces a complete sensory loss with weakness from that level down. The weakness is characteristically caused by a disruption of both the descending motor pathways and the spinal motorneurones. It is typically seen as a part of *multiple sclerosis* or a secondary acute demyelinating process in response to some infection such as an atypical pneumonia.

Brain

Abnormalities in supraspinal sites can result from a variety of causes and depending on the disease process and site determines the type of sensory disturbance. Typically, hemispheric lesions give a loss of sensation down the contralateral side of the body. Brainstem lesions give a range of sensory deficits depending on the exact level of the lesion; thus, pontine lesion can give ipsilateral sensory loss of the face but contralateral sensory loss in the limbs.

Cortical lesions can give a loss of sensation if the primary somatosensory cortex is involved, or can give more complex sensory deficits such as astereognosis (an inability to recognize objects by touch) or even sensory neglect or inattention. These latter abnormalities are typically seen with lesions of the posterior parietal cortex (see Chapter 32).

In some cases, irritative lesions of the primary sensory cortex give rise to simple partial seizures (see Chapter 59) in which the patient experiences brief migrating sensory symptoms up one side of the body. This can also be seen in some patients with transient ischaemic attacks (TIAs).

Pain syndromes can also develop with central lesions and this is best seen in small thalamic vascular events, where dysaesthesia is found in the contralateral limb in a typically diffuse distribution (see Chapter 24).

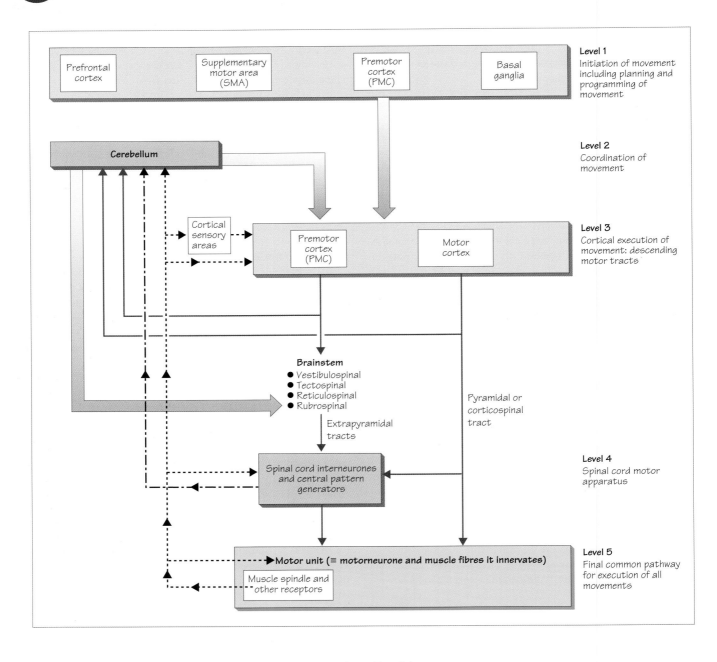

The **motor systems** are those areas of the nervous system that are primarily responsible for controlling movement. The movement can either be guided by inputs from the sensory systems (**closed-loop or reflexly controlled**) or triggered by a sensory cue or some internal desire to move (**open-loop or volitional movement**). In practice, most motor acts involve both types of movement, with closed-loop movements predominantly involving the axial or proximal muscles responsible for balance, posture and locomotion while the open-loop movements are typically associated with the distal musculature concerned with the control of fine skilled movements.

The organization of the motor structures is best viewed in terms of a hierarchy.

Level 1

The highest level of motor control is concerned with the **initiation, planning and programming of movements** in response to an internal desire to move. This desire probably originates in the **limbic system** (see Chapter 46) and **posterior parietal cortex** (see Chapter 32), while the structures primarily responsible for translating that desire into a movement are the **basal ganglia** (see Chapters 40 and 41) and their cortical projection areas in the frontal lobe (see Chapters 37 and 38). These cortical areas include the **supplementary motor area (SMA)** and **premotor cortex (PMC)**; the latter also has a specific role in the control of proximal muscles (see below).

Damage to the basal ganglia and their cortical projection sites leads to a range of complex movement disorders, which includes *Parkinson's disease*, as well as the development of abnormal involuntary movements such as *chorea*, *dystonia* and *ballismus* (see Chapter 41 for the definition of these terms). Damage to these areas does *not* produce any specific weakness or changes in the monosynaptic tendon reflexes (see Chapter 35) but alters the ability to activate or suppress movements.

Level 2

The next level is occupied by the **cerebellum**, which is responsible for the **coordination of movement**. It achieves this by comparing the intended movement descending from the motor areas in the cerebral cortex with the actual movement as detected by the activity of muscle afferents and interneurones (INs) in the spinal cord. It is capable of storing motor information, and this motor memory is not only useful in the learning of new movements but also in the correct timing of muscle activations during complex movements.

Damage to this structure leads primarily to a breakdown in the coordination of movement, without any specific weakness (see Chapter 39).

Level 3

The middle level is concerned with the control of the lower motorneurones (MNs) by the supraspinal **descending motor pathways**. This can broadly be divided into two sets of pathways.

1 The corticospinal (CoST) or pyramidal tract which originates in the motor, premotor and somatosensory cortices and synapses directly on to the MN in the brainstem cranial nerve nuclei and ventral (or anterior) horn of the spinal cord and to a lesser extent INs.

2 The extrapyramidal tracts which originate from subcortical structures and have a more complex distribution of synaptic contacts with both MNs and INs. These extrapyramidal pathways include the vestibulo- (VeST), reticulo- (ReST), tecto- (TeST) and rubrospinal tracts (RuST) and are all in receipt of an input from the primary motor cortex.

Damage in the central nervous system (CNS) is rarely specific to a single tract but interruption of the descending motor pathways produces a pattern of weakness in the limbs that is more pronounced in the extensor muscles in the arms and flexor muscles in the legs—the so-called (but misnamed) **pyramidal distribution of weakness**. In association with the weakness, there is increased tone in the muscles and brisk reflexes; all three features characterizing an ***upper MN lesion*** (see Chapter 43). In contrast to the higher levels in the hierarchy, this is the first level where damage is actually associated with weakness.

Level 4

A low level of motor organization is to be found in the **spinal cord** itself. The descending motor pathways from the brain synapse not only on the MNs but also the INs, and while some of these mediate the spinal cord **reflexes**, others are capable of generating their own outputs to MNs independently of any descending or peripheral sensory input—**central pattern generators**. These are important in locomotion (see Chapter 36), although their existence and role in it humans is still unresolved.

Level 5

The lowest level or **final common pathway of the motor system** is the output neurone of the CNS to the muscle (the **MN**). The MN not only receives information from the brain via the descending pathways and spinal cord INs but also has an important input from sensory organs in the periphery, especially the **muscle spindle** and **Golgi tendon organ** that are found in the muscle and tendon, respectively (see Chapter 35). The muscle spindle in particular is important in mediating the **simple stretch reflex** that underlies the tendon jerks of the clinical examination and is important in maintaining muscle tone.

Damage to the MN or its axon to the muscle produces a *lower* (as opposed to upper) *MN lesion*, characterized by weakness and wasting, hypotonia and reduced or absent reflexes (see Chapters 35 and 43).

A cautionary note

It is important to remember that the division of the CNS into motor and sensory functions is a gross simplification as all the motor areas have some sensory input. It is difficult to know the point at which a highly processed sensory input becomes the impulse for the initiation of a movement. It should also be realized that the division of the motor systems into various levels and different motor pools is a convenient but not strictly accurate device for understanding the control of movement and the pathophysiology of disorders of the motor system.

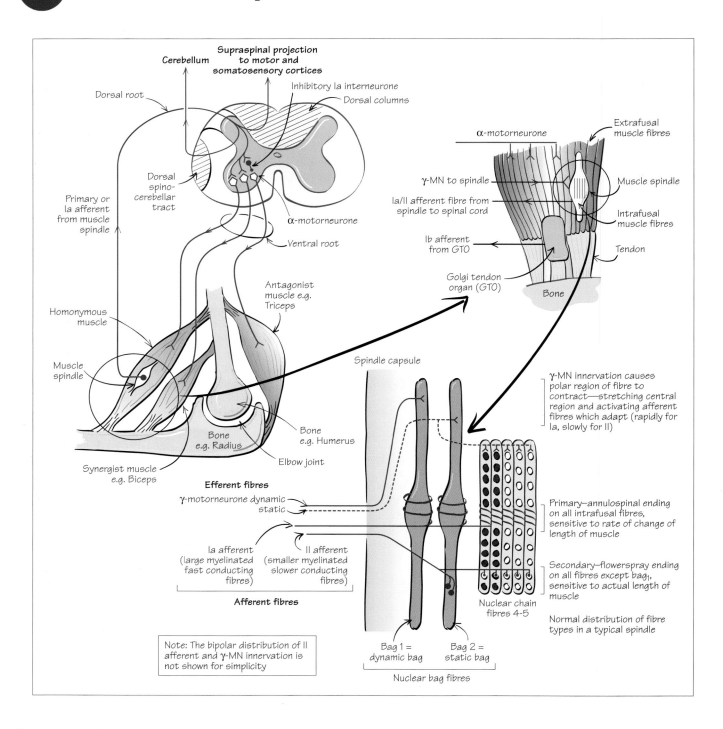

Lower motorneurone

The **lower motorneurone (LMN)** is defined as the neurone whose cell body lies in either the anterior or ventral horn of the spinal cord or cranial nerve nuclei of the brainstem and which directly innervates the muscle via its axon. The number of muscle fibres innervated by a single axon is termed the **motor unit**. The smaller the number of fibres per motorneurone (MN) axon, the finer the control (e.g. the extraocular muscles).

The MNs of the anterior horn are divided into two types: the **α-MN** (70 μm in diameter) which innervate the muscle itself (the force generating extrafusal fibres); and the **γ-MN** (30 μm in diameter) which innervate the intrafusal fibres of the muscle spindle. The **muscle spindle** is an encapsulated sense organ found within the muscle, which is responsible for detecting the extent of muscle contraction by monitoring the length of muscle fibres.

It is the muscle spindle and its connections to the spinal cord that mediates the **tendon reflexes**; sudden stretching of a muscle by a sharp tap of a tendon hammer transiently activates the **Ia afferent nerve endings** which, via an excitatory monosynaptic input to the MN, causes that muscle (the **homonymous muscle**) to contract briefly (e.g. the knee jerk). In addition, the Ia afferent input from the muscle spindle, while activating other **synergistic muscles** with a similar action to the homonymous muscle, also inhibits muscles with opposing actions (**antagonist muscles**) through a Ia inhibitory interneurone (IN) in the spinal cord. However, it must be stressed that tendon jerks reflect not only the integrity of this circuit but the overall excitability of the MN, which is increased in cases of an upper MN lesion (see Chapter 43).

Muscle spindle

The **muscle spindle** lies in parallel to the extrafusal muscle fibres and consists of the following.

• **Nuclear bag and chain fibres** which have different morphological properties: the bag 1 or dynamic fibres are very sensitive to the rate of change in muscle length, while the bag 2 or static bag fibres are like the nuclear chain fibres in being more sensitive to the absolute length of the muscle.

• A **γ-MN** that synapses at the polar ends of the intrafusal muscle fibres and which can be one of two types: **dynamic or static**, with the latter innervating all but the bag 1 fibres. Both types of γ-MN are usually coactivated with the α-MN so that the intrafusal fibres contract at the same time as do the extrafusal fibres, thus ensuring that the spindle maintains its sensitivity during muscle contraction. Occasionally, the γ-MN can be activated independently of the α-MN, typically when the animal is learning some new complex movement, which increases the sensitivity of the spindle to changes in length.

• Two types of afferent fibres and nerve endings: a **Ia afferent fibre** associated with an annulospiral nerve ending winding around the centre of all types of intrafusal fibres (**primary ending**); and a slower conducting **type II fibre** which is associated with flowerspray endings on the more polar regions of the intrafusal fibres (with the exception of the bag 1 fibres; the **secondary ending**). The stretching of the intrafusal fibre activates both types of fibre. However, the Ia fibre is most sensitive to the rate of change in fibre length, while the type II fibres respond more to the overall length of the fibre rather than the rate of change in fibre length.

The spindle relays via the dorsal root to a number of central nervous system (CNS) sites including: (i) the MNs innervating the homonymous and synergistic muscles (the basis of the stretch reflex); (ii) INs inhibiting the antagonist muscles; (iii) the cerebellum via the dorsal spinocerebellar tract; (iv) the somatosensory cortex; and (v) the primary motor cortex via the dorsal column–medial lemniscal pathways. Thus, the muscle spindle is not only responsible for mediating simple stretch or tendon reflexes and through this muscle tone but is also involved in the coordination of movement, the perception of joint position (proprioception) and the modulation of long-latency or transcortical reflexes (see Chapter 38).

Damage to the spindle afferent fibres (e.g. in large fibre *neuropathies*) produces hypotonia (as the stretch reflex is important in controlling the normal tone of muscles), incoordination, reduced joint position sense and, occasionally, tremor with an inability to learn new motor skills in the face of novel environmental situations. In addition, large fibre neuropathies disrupt other somatosensory afferent inputs (see Chapters 22 and 33).

The **Golgi tendon organ** is found at the junction between muscle and tendon and thus lies in series with the extrafusal muscle fibres. It monitors the degree of muscle contraction in terms of the muscular force generated and relays this to the spinal cord via a **Ib afferent fibre**. This sensory organ, in addition to providing useful information to the CNS on the degree of tension within muscles, serves to prevent excessive muscular contractions (see Chapter 36). Thus, when activated it inhibits the agonist muscle.

Motorneurone recruitment and damage

The **'principle of recruitment'** corresponds to the order in which different types of muscle fibres are activated. The smallest α-MNs, which are those most easily excited by any input, innervate type 1 (*not* to be confused with the bag 1 intrafusal fibres found in the spindle) or slow-contracting fibres which are responsible for increasing and maintaining the tension in a muscle.

The next population of MNs to be activated are those that innervate the type 2A or fast-contracting/resistant to fatigue fibres which are responsible for virtually all forms of locomotion. Finally, the largest MNs are only activated by maximal inputs, which innervate type 2B or fast-contracting/easily fatigued fibres that are responsible for running or jumping.

The order of recruitment of MNs to a given input follows a simple relationship known as the **size principle**, which allows muscles to contract in a logical sequence.

The **α-MN itself can be damaged** in a number of different conditions but in all cases the clinical features are the same; there is wasting of the denervated muscles with weakness, and reduced or absent reflexes (a lower MN lesion). In some cases one can also see fasciculations (muscle twitchings), as the loss of the motorneuronal input to the muscle leads to a more random redistribution of the acetylcholine receptors away from sites of the old neuromuscular junction.

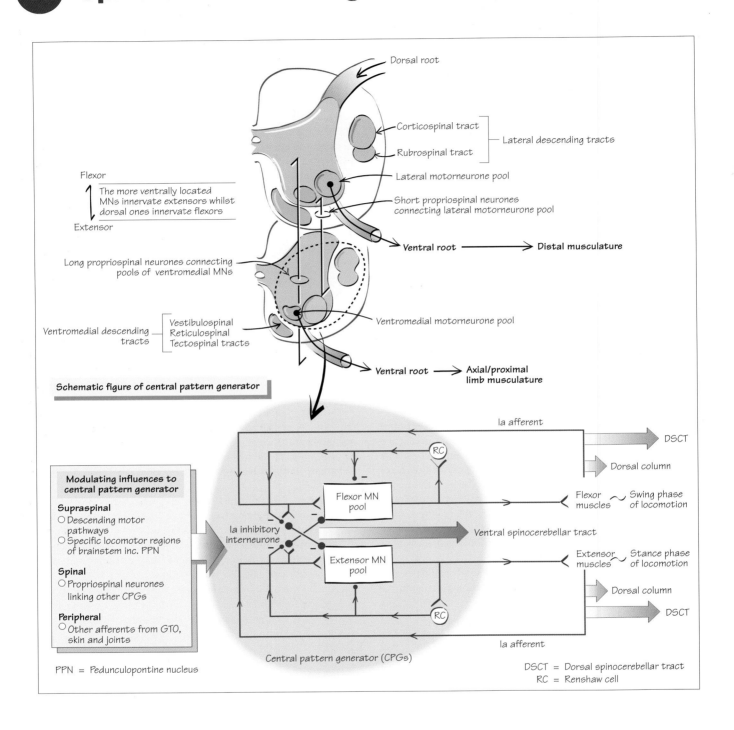

Schematic figure of central pattern generator

Flexor
↑ The more ventrally located MNs innervate extensors whilst dorsal ones innervate flexors
Extensor

Dorsal root

Corticospinal tract
Rubrospinal tract — Lateral descending tracts

Lateral motorneurone pool
Short propriospinal neurones connecting lateral motorneurone pool

Ventral root → Distal musculature

Long propriospinal neurones connecting pools of ventromedial MNs

Ventromedial descending tracts — Vestibulospinal / Reticulospinal / Tectospinal tracts

Ventromedial motorneurone pool

Ventral root → Axial/proximal limb musculature

Modulating influences to central pattern generator

Supraspinal
○ Descending motor pathways
○ Specific locomotor regions of brainstem inc. PPN

Spinal
○ Propriospinal neurones linking other CPGs

Peripheral
○ Other afferents from GTO, skin and joints

PPN = Pedunculopontine nucleus

Ia afferent
DSCT
Dorsal column
Flexor MN pool
Flexor muscles ~ Swing phase of locomotion
Ia inhibitory interneurone
Ventral spinocerebellar tract
Extensor MN pool
Extensor muscles ~ Stance phase of locomotion
Dorsal column
DSCT
Ia afferent

Central pattern generator (CPGs)

DSCT = Dorsal spinocerebellar tract
RC = Renshaw cell

Spinal cord motor organization

In addition to containing the **α- and γ-motorneurones (MNs)**, the spinal cord also contains a large number of **interneurones (INs)** which relay afferent information from the periphery and supraspinal sites. These INs can form networks that are intrinsically active and whose output governs the activity of MNs, **central pattern generators (CPGs)**. These CPGs, which may underlie locomotion, while not requiring any afferent input in order to produce a patterned motor output, are nevertheless modulated by both central and peripheral inputs (see Chapters 35 and 37). Such CPGs are not unique to locomotion as they can be seen in other parts of the CNS controlling rhythmical motor activities, e.g. respiration and the brainstem respiratory network.

Descending motor pathways

(see Appendix 2b for details of individual tracts)

The **descending motor pathways** can be classified according to:
- their site of origin, namely pyramidal or extrapyramidal tracts (although *clinically extrapyramidal disorders* refer to diseases of the basal ganglia; see Chapter 40); or
- their location within the cord and the muscles they ultimately innervate through the MNs.

Thus, the **pyramidal (corticospinal)** and **rubrospinal tract** are associated with a **lateral MN pool** that innervates the distal musculature, while the **vestibulo-, reticulo- and tectospinal tracts** are more associated with a **ventromedial MN pool** that innervates the axial and proximal musculature.

These latter MNs are linked by long **propriospinal neurones**, while the converse is true for the lateral MN pool. Thus, the **lateral motor system** is more involved in the control of fine distal movements, while the **ventromedial system** is more concerned with balance and posture.

The MNs of the anterior horn are further organized such that the most ventrally located MNs innervate the extensor muscles, while those found at more dorsal locations innervate the flexor musculature.

Locomotion

The control of **locomotion** is complex, as it requires the coordinated movement of all four limbs in most mammals.

Each cycle in locomotion is termed a **step** and involves a **stance** and a **swing** phase—the latter being that part of the cycle when the foot is not in contact with the ground. Each cycle requires the correct sequential activation of flexors and extensors. The simplest way to achieve this is to have **two CPGs (half centres)** which activate flexors and extensors, respectively, and which mutually inhibit each other.

This mutual inhibition can perhaps best be modelled using the **inhibitory Ia IN** and **Renshaw cells**. Renshaw cells are INs that, when activated by MNs, inhibit those same MNs (see Chapter 8). Thus, the activation of an MN pool by a CPG leads to its own inhibition and the removal of an inhibitory input to the antagonistic CPG, thus switching the muscle groups activated. This half centre model for locomotion can be modulated by a range of descending and peripheral inputs. In this latter respect the Ib afferent from the Golgi tendon organ (GTO) can switch the CPGs to prevent excessive tension developing in a muscle, while a range of cutaneous inputs can cause the cycle to be modified in the event of an obstacle being encountered. These afferents, termed **flexor reflex afferents**, cause the limb to be flexed so stepping over or withdrawing from the noxious or obstructive object.

CPGs within the spinal cord communicate with each other through propriospinal neurones. In contrast, supraspinal communication of information from and about the CPGs is relayed indirectly in the form of muscle spindle Ia afferent activity via the dorsal spinocerebellar tract (DSCT) and dorsal columns and spinal cord interneuronal activity via the ventral spinocerebellar tract (VSCT).

Clinical disorders of spinal cord motor control and locomotion

Although experimental animals can locomote in the absence of any significant supraspinal inputs (**fictive locomotion**), this is not the case in humans. However, clinical disorders of gait are relatively common and may occur for a number of reasons.

Disorders of spinal cord INs such as occurs in *stiff-person syndrome* are rare. In this condition the patient presents with increased tone or rigidity in the axial muscles ± spasms caused by the continuous firing of the MNs as a result of the loss of an inhibitory interneuronal input primarily to the ventromedial MNs. This condition is associated with antibodies against the synthetic enzyme for γ-aminobutyric acid (GABA), glutamic acid decarboxylase (GAD), although it is still not clear whether these antibodies are pathogenic in this disorder.

Damage to the descending pathways can produce a range of deficiencies. The most devastating is that seen with extensive brainstem damage when there is uninhibited extensor muscle activity and the patient adopts a characteristic *decerebrate posture* with arching of the neck and back and rigid extension of all four limbs. In contrast, a more rostrally placed lesion in one of the cerebral hemispheres produces weakness down the contralateral side (hemiplegia or hemiparesis) with increased tone (hypertonia) and increased tendon reflexes (hyperreflexia) which may produce spontaneous or stretch-induced rhythmic involuntary muscular contractions (clonus). This situation is also seen with interruption of the descending motor pathways in the spinal cord (see Chapters 33, 34 and 43).

The pattern of weakness in such lesions characteristically involves the extensors more than the flexors in the upper limb and the converse in the lower limb. This is misleadingly termed a **pyramidal distribution of weakness**, as damage confined to the pyramidal tract in monkeys leads only to a deficiency in fine finger movements with a degree of hypotonia and hypo- or areflexia.

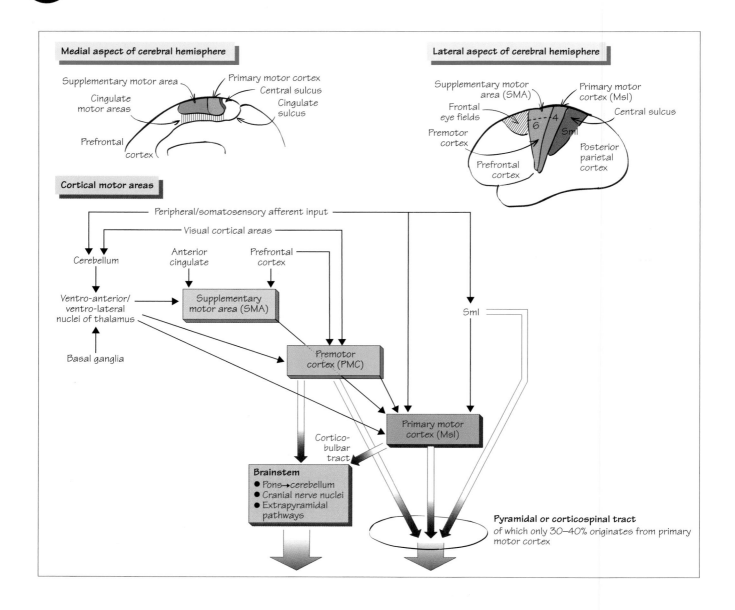

There are a number of cortical areas involved with the control of movement including the primary motor cortex (see Chapter 38), premotor cortex (PMC), supplementary motor area (SMA) and a number of adjacent areas in the anterior cingulate cortex. In addition, there are other areas that have specific roles in the cortical control of movement, including the frontal eye fields (see Chapter 42) and posterior parietal cortex (see Chapter 32). This chapter briefly discusses the organization of the motor cortical areas and their relative roles in movement control, while the next chapter concentrates on the primary motor cortex.

Primary motor cortex

The **primary motor cortex (MsI)** is that part of the cerebral cortex that produces a motor response with the minimum electrical stimulation. It corresponds to Brodmann's area 4 and lies just in front of the central sulcus and projects to the motorneurones (MNs) of the brain-stem via the **corticobulbar tracts** and to the MNs of the spinal cord directly via the **corticospinal tract (CoST)** and indirectly via the sub-cortical extrapyramidal tracts. Indeed, MsI is particularly closely associated with the pyramidal tract (even though 60–70% of it originates in other cortical areas) and so has a role in the control of distal muscula-ture and fine movements (see Chapters 36 and 38).

Other cortical areas

A range of other cortical areas are involved in the control of movement, including the **PMC** (corresponding to the lateral part of Brodmann's area 6); the **SMA** (corresponding to the medial aspect of Brodmann's area 6); a number of motor areas centred on the **anterior cingulate cortex** on the medial aspect of the frontal lobe; the **frontal eye fields** (corresponding to Brodmann's area 8); and the **posterior parietal cortex** (especially Brodmann's area 7).

Some of these areas have specialist functions such as the frontal eye fields with eye movement control (see Chapter 42) and the posterior parietal cortex with the visual control of movement (see Chapter 32). The remaining areas in the frontal lobe are involved with more complex aspects of movement. Most of these other cortical areas therefore occupy a higher level in the motor hierarchy than MsI, and their connections and functions are summarized in the figure and Table 37.1 (see also Chapter 34).

The PMC refers to a specific area of Brodmann's area 6, and like the primary motor cortex has an input directly to the spinal MNs via the corticospinal or pyramidal tract. This area therefore occupies two levels of the motor hierarchy as it also has a role in the planning of movement (see Chapter 34). In contrast, the SMA lies medial to the PMC, and has a much more clearly defined role in the planning of movements especially in response to sensory cues. Furthermore, it is now clear that the SMA is part of a much larger number of higher order motor cortical areas that lie along the medial side of the frontal cortex and which are involved in the planning of movements more than their execution. It is these cortical areas that receive the predominant outflow of the basal ganglia (see Chapter 40), which helps explain the abnormal movements that are seen with diseases of this area of the brain (see Chapter 41). For example, in **Parkinson's disease** there is a slowness and poverty of movement that is associated with underactivation of these cortical areas, a situation that is rectified by the administration of antiparkinsonian medication or successful neurosurgical interventions.

Table 37.1 Cortical motor areas: connections and functions.

Cortical area	Afferent input	Efferent output	Neurophysiology	Function

Primary motor cortex (MsI)	SMA
	PMC
	SmI
	Cerebellum via thalamus (VA–VL nuclei)
	
	Dorsal column–medial lemniscal system (VP via nucleus of thalamus)
		Corticospinal or pyramidal tract
		Brainstem:
		  Pons to cerebellum
		  Cranial nerve nuclei
		  Extrapyramidal tracts
			Lesion of MsI results in a loss of placing, hopping reactions and skilled manipulative movements	Control of distal musculature and fine skilled movements
				Role in reflex control of movement (transcortical reflexes)

Premotor cortex (PMC)	SMA
	Prefrontal cortex
	Somatosensory and visual cortices
	Cerebellum via thalamus (VA–VL nuclei)
	Basal ganglia via thalamus (VA–VL nuclei)
		MsI
		Corticospinal or pyramidal tract
		Brainstem:
		  pons to cerebellum
		  extrapyramidal pathways
			Lesion of PMC produces a mild paresis and impairment of skilled movements; deficits in executing visuomotor tasks
			Regional blood flow studies show it is activated during tasks requiring directional guidance of a movement from sensory information
				Control of proximal musculature
				Control of movement sequence and preparation for movement

Supplementary motor area (SMA)	Prefrontal cortex Basal ganglia via thalamus (VA–VL nuclei) Anterior cingulate cortex Contralateral SMA	SMA (contralateral) PMC MsI	Lesion of SMA produces a severe reduction in spontaneous motor activity with forced grasping and failure of bimanual coordination Stimulation of SMA produces vocalization and complex bilateral arm movements Activity in SMA precedes any changes in MsI Units in SMA respond maximally to sensory cues being used as an instruction for a movement Regional blood-flow studies have shown an increased flow with the planning or thinking of a motor act	Role in the initiation and planning of movement Role in bimanual coordination

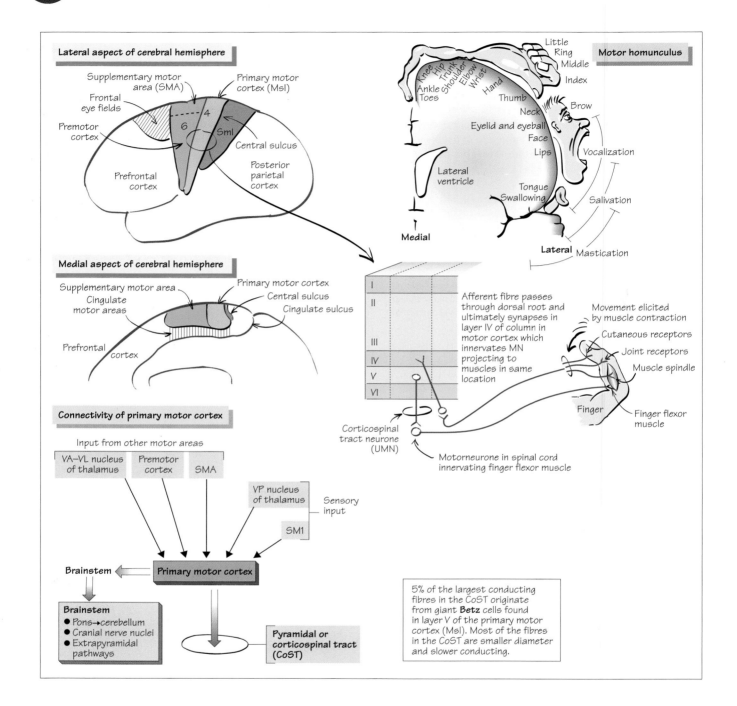

The primary motor cortex (MsI) receives afferent information from the cerebellum (via the thalamus) and more anteriorly placed motor cortical areas such as the supplementary motor area (SMA) and a sensory input from the muscle spindle as well as cortical sensory areas. This latter sensory input emphasizes the artificial way in which the central nervous system (CNS) is divided up into motor and sensory systems and in order to acknowledge this the primary motor cortex is termed the MsI while the primary somatosensory cortex is termed the SmI (see Chapter 22).

Investigation of the **organization of MsI** has shown that the motor innervation of the body is organized in a highly topographical fashion, with the cortical representation of each body part being proportional to the degree of motor innervation—so, for example, the hand and oro-buccal musculature have a large cortical representation. The resultant distorted image of the body in MsI is known as the **motor homunculus**, with the head represented laterally and the feet medially.

This organization may be manifest clinically in patients with *epilepsy* that originates in the motor cortex. In such cases the epileptic fit may begin at one site, typically the hand, and then spread so that the jerking marches out from the site of origin (**Jacksonian march**, named after the neurologist, Hughlings Jackson). This is in contrast to the clinical picture seen with seizures arising from the SMA, in which the patient raises both arms and vocalizes with complex repetitive movements suggesting that this area has a higher role in motor control (see Chapter 38).

These studies on the motor homunculus by Penfield and colleagues in the 1950s revealed the macroscopic organization of MsI, but subsequent microelectrode studies in animals revealed that MsI is composed of **cortical columns** (see Chapter 15). The inputs to a column consist of afferent fibres from the joint, muscle spindle and skin which are maximally activated by contraction of those muscles innervated by that same area of cortex. So, for example, a group of cortical columns in MsI will receive sensory inputs from a finger when it is flexed—that input being provided by the skin receptors on the front of the finger, the muscle spindles in the finger flexors and the joint receptors of the finger joints. That same column will also send a projection to the motorneurones (MNs) in the spinal cord that innervate the finger flexors. Activation of the corticospinal neurone from that column will ultimately activate the receptors that project to that same column, and vice versa. Thus, each column is said to have **input–output coupling** and this may be important in the more complex reflex control of movement as, for example, with the **long-latency or transcortical reflexes**. These reflexes refer to the delayed and smaller electromyographical (EMG) changes that are seen following the sudden stretch of a muscle—the first EMG change being the M1 response of the monosynaptic stretch reflex (see Chapter 35). The transcortical reflex has as its afferent limb

the muscle spindle input via the Ia fibre (relayed via the dorsal column–medial lemniscal pathway) and the efferent pathway involves the corticospinal tract (CoST). The exact role of this reflex is not known but it may be important in controlling movements precisely, especially when unexpected obstacles are encountered which activate the muscle spindle.

There has been great controversy as to whether MsI controls individual muscles, simple movements or some other aspect of movements. Neurones within MsI fire before any EMG changes and appear to **code for the direction and force of a movement**, although this activity is dependent on the nature of the task being performed. Therefore, as a whole, the motor cortex controls movement by its innervation of populations of MNs, as individual corticospinal axons innervate many different MNs.

MsI is capable of being remodelled after lesions or changes in sensory feedback, implying that it maintains a flexible relationship with the muscles throughout life. Thus, cells in a region of MsI can shift from the control of one set of muscles to a new set. Within given areas of cortex there is some evidence that synaptic strengths can be altered with long-term potentiation (see Chapter 46), which suggests that the MsI may be capable of learning new movements, a function traditionally ascribed to the cerebellum (see Chapter 39).

Damage to MsI in isolation is rare and experimentally tends to produce deficiencies similar to those seen with selective pyramidal tract lesions. However, damage to both MsI and adjacent premotor areas, as occurs in most *cerebrovascular accidents (CVAs)* involving the middle cerebral artery (see Chapter 19), produces a much more significant deficiency, with a significant hemiparesis.

39 The cerebellum

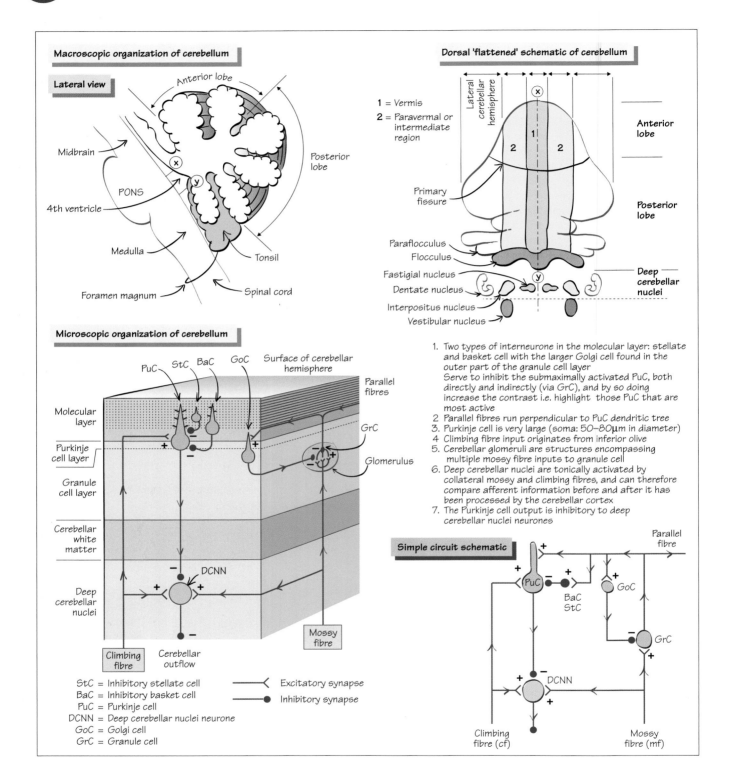

Macroscopic organization of cerebellum

Lateral view

Anterior lobe
Midbrain
PONS
4th ventricle
Medulla
Foramen magnum
Posterior lobe
Tonsil
Spinal cord

Dorsal 'flattened' schematic of cerebellum

1 = Vermis
2 = Paravermal or intermediate region

Lateral cerebellar hemisphere

Anterior lobe

Primary fissure

Posterior lobe

Paraflocculus
Flocculus
Fastigial nucleus
Dentate nucleus
Interpositus nucleus
Vestibular nucleus

Deep cerebellar nuclei

Microscopic organization of cerebellum

PuC StC BaC GoC Surface of cerebellar hemisphere

Molecular layer
Purkinje cell layer
Granule cell layer
Cerebellar white matter
Deep cerebellar nuclei

Parallel fibres
GrC
Glomerulus
DCNN
Climbing fibre
Cerebellar outflow
Mossy fibre

StC = Inhibitory stellate cell
BaC = Inhibitory basket cell
PuC = Purkinje cell
DCNN = Deep cerebellar nuclei neurone
GoC = Golgi cell
GrC = Granule cell

Excitatory synapse
Inhibitory synapse

1. Two types of interneurone in the molecular layer: stellate and basket cell with the larger Golgi cell found in the outer part of the granule cell layer
   Serve to inhibit the submaximally activated PuC, both directly and indirectly (via GrC), and by so doing increase the contrast i.e. highlight those PuC that are most active
2. Parallel fibres run perpendicular to PuC dendritic tree
3. Purkinje cell is very large (soma: 50–80µm in diameter)
4. Climbing fibre input originates from inferior olive
5. Cerebellar glomeruli are structures encompassing multiple mossy fibre inputs to granule cell
6. Deep cerebellar nuclei are tonically activated by collateral mossy and climbing fibres, and can therefore compare afferent information before and after it has been processed by the cerebellar cortex
7. The Purkinje cell output is inhibitory to deep cerebellar nuclei neurones

Simple circuit schematic

Parallel fibre
PuC
BaC StC
GoC
GrC
DCNN
Climbing fibre (cf)
Mossy fibre (mf)

Organization of the cerebellum

The **cerebellum (CBM)** is a complex structure found below the tentorial membrane in the posterior fossa and connected to the brainstem by three pairs of (cerebellar) peduncles (see Chapter 13). It is primarily involved in the coordination and learning of movements, and is best thought of in terms of three functional and anatomical systems:

1 spinoCBM—involved with the control of axial musculature and posture ▓ + ▪;

2 pontoCBM—involved with the coordination and planning of limb movements □; and

3 vestibuloCBM—involved with posture and the control of eye movements ▨.

These three systems have their own unique pattern of connections (see Appendix 3). The spinoCBM can be divided into a vermal and paravermal (intermediate) region with the former having a close association with the axial musculature. It is therefore associated with the ventromedial descending motor pathways and motorneurones (MNs) while the paravermal part of the spinoCBM is more concerned with the coordination of the limbs. The pontoCBM has a role in this coordination but is more concerned with the visual control of movement by relaying information from the posterior parietal cortex to the motor cortical areas. The vestibuloCBM has no associated deep cerebellar nucleus and is phylogenetically one of the oldest parts of the cerebellum. It, like the vermal part of the spinoCBM, is more concerned with balance through its connections with the ventromedial motor pathways but also has a role in the control of eye movements (see Chapter 42).

In general, the CBM compares the intended movement originating from the motor cortical areas with the actual movement as relayed by the muscle afferents and spinal cord interneurones while receiving an important input from the vestibular and visual system. The comparison having been made, an error signal is relayed via descending motor pathways, and the correction factor stored as part of a motor memory in the synaptic inputs to the Purkinje cell (PuC). This modifiable synapse at the level of the PuC is an example of **long-term depression** (LTD; see Chapters 47 and 50). It describes the reduced synaptic input of the parallel fibre (pf) to PuC when it is activated in phase and at low frequency with the climbing fibre input to that same PuC and persists for several hours at least. In other words, at times of new movements the climbing fibre input to the PuC increases which has a modifying effect on the pf input to that same PuC. As the movement becomes more routine, the climbing fibre (cf) lessens but the modified (reduced) pf input persists: it is this modification that is thought to underlie the learning and memory of movements.

This modifiable synapse was first proposed by Marr in 1969 and subsequently has been verified, especially with respect to the vestibulo-ocular reflex (see Chapters 30 and 50). The biochemical basis of LTD in the CBM is unknown but appears to rely on the activation of different glutamate receptors in the PuC and the subsequent influx of calcium and the activation of a protein kinase. The presence of a modifiable synapse implies that the CBM is capable of learning and storing information in a motor memory (see Appendix 3).

The microscopic organization of the cerebellum, which allows for the generation of LTD, is well characterized even if the biochemical basis for it remains obscure. The excitatory input to the cerebellum is provided by a mossy and climbing fibre input. The mossy fibre indirectly activates PuC through pfs that originate from granule cells (GrC). In contrast, the climbing fibre directly synapses on the PuC and, as with the mossy fibre input, there is an input to the deep cerebellar nuclei neurones (DCNN). These neurones are therefore tonically excited by the input fibres to the cerebellum, and are inhibited by the output from the cerebellar cortex (the PuC). The PuC in turn are inhibited by a number of local interneurones, while Golgi cells (GoC) in the outer granule cell layer provide an inhibitory input to the GrC. All of these interneurones have the effect of inhibiting submaximally activated PuC and GrC, and by so doing highlight the signal to be analysed.

The final output of the cerebellum from the deep cerebellar nuclei to various brainstem structures is also inhibitory.

Clinical features of cerebellar damage

Much that can be deduced about the function of the CBM is derived from the clinical features of patients with cerebellar damage.

Dysfunction of the CBM is found in a large number of conditions, and the clinical features of cerebellar damage are as follow.

1 Hypotonia or reduced muscle tone. This is caused by a reduced input from the DCNN via the descending motor pathways to the muscle spindle (see Chapter 35).

2 Incoordination/ataxia. There are a number of manifestations of this including: asynergy (an inability to coordinate the contraction of agonist and antagonist muscles); dysmetria (an inability to terminate movements accurately which can result in an intention tremor and past pointing); and dysdiadochokinesis (an inability to perform rapidly alternating movements). Ataxia is often used to describe incoordinated movements. In cases where the vermis is predominantly involved, as occurs in alcoholic cerebellar degeneration, this results in a staggering, wide-based, 'drunk-like' character to the gait. When there is involvement of the more lateral parts of the cerebellar hemisphere the incoordination involves the limbs.

3 Dysarthria. This is an inability to articulate words properly caused by incoordination of the oropharyngeal musculature. The words are slurred and spoken slowly (scanning dysarthia).

4 Nystagmus. This describes rapid jerky eye movements caused by a breakdown in the outflow from the vestibular nucleus and its connections with the oculomotor nuclei (see Chapters 30 and 42).

5 Palatal tremor or myoclonus. This is a rare condition in which there is hypertrophy of the inferior olive, with damage in a triangle bounded by this structure, the dentate nucleus of the CBM and the red nucleus in the midbrain (Mollaret triangle). The patient characteristically has a low-frequency tremor of the palate, which oscillates up and down.

Finally, there is a recent suggestion that the cerebellum may also subserve some cognitive function as subtle deficits can be seen in this domain in some patients with cerebellar disease.

Function of the cerebellum

The **role of the CBM** can be defined by area and correlates well with the localizing signs of cerebellar disease. Exactly how the CBM achieves these functions is unknown, but the repetition of the same elementary circuitry in all parts of the cerebellar cortex implies a common mode of function. Three possibilities exist which are not mutually exclusive.

1 By acting as a comparator. The CBM compares the descending supraspinal motor signals (efference copy, intended movement) with the ascending afferent feedback information (actual movement), and any discrepancy is corrected by the output of the CBM through descending motor pathways. This allows the CBM to coordinate movements so that they are achieved smoothly and accurately.

2 By acting as a timing device. The CBM (especially the pontoCBM) converts descending motor signals into a sequence of motor activation so that movement is performed in a smooth and coordinated fashion, with balance and posture maintained by the vestibulo- and spinoCBM.

3 By initiating and storing movements. The existence of a modifiable synapse at the level of the PuC means that the CBM is capable of storing motor information and updating it. Therefore, under the appropriate circumstances, the right sequence for a movement can be accessed and fed through the supraspinal motor pathways, and by so doing initiate an accurate learnt movement (see also Chapter 47).

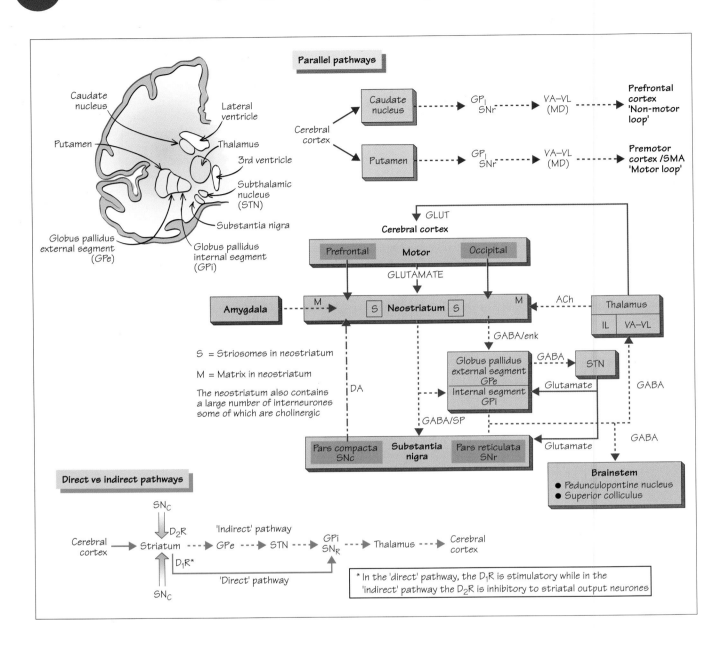

The **basal ganglia** consist of the **caudate and putamen (dorsal or neostriatum; NS)**, the **internal and external segments of the globus pallidus (GPi and GPe,** respectively), the **pars reticulata and pars compacta of the substantia nigra (SNr and SNc,** respectively) and the **subthalamic nucleus (STN)**.

The NS is the main receiving area of the basal ganglia and receives information from the whole cortex in a somatotopic fashion as well as the intralaminar nuclei of the thalamus (IL). The major outflow from the basal ganglia is via the GPi and SNr to the ventroanterior–ventrolateral nuclei of the thalamus (VA–VL) which in turn project to the premotor cortex (PMC), supplementary motor area (SMA) and prefrontal cortex. In addition, there is a projection to the brainstem, especially to the pedunculopontine nucleus (PPN) that is involved in locomotion (see Chapter 36), and to the superior colliculus that is involved with eye movements (see Chapters 26 and 42).

The basal ganglia also have a **number of loops** within them that are important. There is a striato–nigral–striatal loop with the latter projection being dopaminergic in nature. This pathway degenerates in **Parkinson's disease**. There is also a loop from the GPe to the STN which then projects back to the GPi and SNr. This pathway is excitatory in nature and is important in controlling the level of activation of the inhibitory output nuclei of the basal ganglia to the thalamus. However, although a marked degree of convergence and divergence can be seen throughout the basal ganglia, the projections do form parallel pathways, which at the most simplistic level divide into a motor pathway through the putamen and a non-motor pathway through the caudate nucleus.

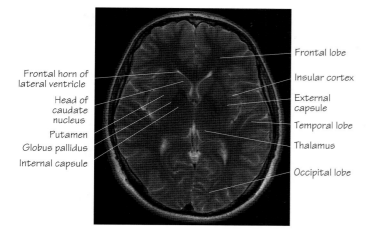

Frontal horn of lateral ventricle

Head of caudate nucleus

Putamen

Globus pallidus

Internal capsule

Frontal lobe

Insular cortex

External capsule

Temporal lobe

Thalamus

Occipital lobe

The NS consists of **patches or striosomes** that are deficient in the enzyme acetylcholinesterase (AChE). These are embedded in an otherwise AChE-rich striatum, which forms the large extrastriosomal **matrix**. In general, the striosomes are closely related to the dopaminergic nigrostriatal pathway and prefrontal cortex and amygdala, while the matrix is more involved with sensorimotor areas. However, the relationship of these two components of the neostriatum to any parallel pathways is not clear.

This non-motor role of the basal ganglia is perhaps more clearly seen with the **ventral extension of the basal ganglia** which consists of the ventral striatum (nucleus accumbens), ventral pallidum and substantia innominata (not shown in the figure). It receives a dopaminergic input from the ventral tegmental area that lies adjacent to the SNc in the midbrain, and projects via the thalamus to the prefrontal cortex and frontal eye fields. These structures are intimately associated with motivation and drug addiction.

The **neurophysiology** of the basal ganglia shows that many of the cells within it have complex properties that are not clearly sensory or motor in terms of their response characteristics. For example, some units in the NS respond to sensory stimuli but only when that sensory stimulus is a trigger for a movement. In contrast, many units in the pallidum respond maximally to movement about a given joint before any electromyographic (EMG) changes. Thus, from a neurophysiological point of view, the basal ganglia take highly processed sensory information and convert it into some form of motor programme. This is supported by the clinical disorders that affect the basal ganglia (see Chapters 41 and 43).

Basal ganglia diseases and their treatment

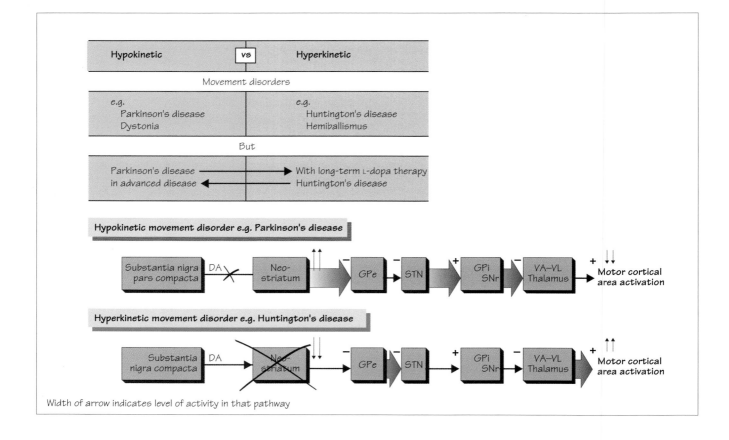

Width of arrow indicates level of activity in that pathway

Parkinson's disease

Parkinson's disease is a degenerative disorder that typically affects people in their sixth and seventh decades of life. The primary pathological event is the loss of the dopaminergic nigrostriatal tract, with the formation of characteristic histological inclusion bodies, known as Lewy bodies. In the vast majority of cases the disease develops for reasons that are not clear (idiopathic Parkinson's disease; see Chapter 57). However, in some cases clear aetiological agents are identified such as vascular lesions in the region of the nigrostriatal pathway, administration of the antidopaminergic drugs in schizophrenia (see Chapter 55) or genetic abnormalities in young patients and some rare families.

Over 50–60% of the dopaminergic nigrostriatal neurones need to be lost before the classical clinical features of idiopathic Parkinson's disease are clearly manifest: slowness to move (bradykinesia); increased tone in the muscles (cogwheel rigidity); and tremor that is present at rest. However, most patients also display a range of cognitive, affective and autonomic abnormalities, which may relate to pathological changes at sites other than the nigrostriatal tract (see also Chapters 47 and 48).

Neurophysiologically, these patients have increased activity of the neurones in the globus pallidus internal segment (GPi) with a disturbed pattern of discharge, which results from increased activity in the subthalamic nucleus (STN) secondary to the loss of the predominantly inhibitory dopaminergic input to the neostriatum (NS). The increased

inhibitory output from the GPi (and presumably the substantia nigra pars reticulata [SNr] as well) to the ventroanterior–ventrolateral nuclei of the thalamus (VA–VL) results in reduced activation of the supplementary motor area (SMA) and other adjacent cortical areas. Thus, patients with Parkinson's disease are unable to initiate movement because of their failure to activate the SMA, although the explanation for the tremor and rigidity is less clear. However, these patients can be treated successfully in the early stages of the disease with various drugs.

Antiparkinsonian drugs

No drug currently has been shown definitely to slow the progression of Parkinson's disease. For most patients, **dopamine replacement therapy** with **levodopa** (L-dopa) or dopamine agonists is the treatment of choice (dopamine itself does not pass the blood–brain barrier). L-dopa is the immediate precursor of dopamine and is converted in the brain by decarboxylation to dopamine. Orally administered L-dopa is largely metabolized outside the brain and so it is given with an extracerebral decarboxylase inhibitor (carbidopa or benserazide), which greatly reduces the effective dose and peripheral adverse effects (e.g. hypotension, nausea). L-dopa frequently produces adverse effects that are mainly caused by widespread stimulation of dopamine receptors. They include nausea and vomiting (as a result of stimulation of the chemoreceptor trigger zone), psychiatric side-effects (e.g. hallucinations, confusion) and dyskinesias. After 5 years' treatment about half of the patients will experience some of these complications. In some the akinesia gradually recurs producing so-called wearing off effects, while in others various dyskinesias may appear in response to L-dopa (so-called L-dopa-induced dyskinesias). These latter problems may lead to rapid changes in the motor state of the individual ('on–off' problems) and is universally found in all cases of advanced Parkinson's disease.

Selegiline and **rasagiline** are selective monoamine oxidase type B (MAO$_B$) inhibitors that reduce the metabolism of dopamine in the brain and potentiate the action of L-dopa. They may be used in conjunction with L-dopa to reduce 'end of dose' deterioration.

Catecholamine-*O*-methyltransferase (COMT) inhibitors such as **entacapone** and **Tolcapone** have recently been developed for use in Parkinson's disease, and they reduce the peripheral metabolism of L-dopa and by so doing increase the amount that can enter the brain.

Dopamine agonists (e.g. ropinirole, cabergoline, pramipexole) are also used often as first-line treatment in young patients or in combination with L-dopa in the later stages of Parkinson's disease in older patients. Dopamine agonists directly bind to the dopamine receptors in the striatum (and substantia nigra) and by so doing activate the post-synaptic output neurones of the striatum. These agents are preferred as the treatment of choice in young-onset Parkinson's disease because of their L-dopa sparing effects which may delay the development of 'on–off' effects, although they are slightly less efficacious in terms of their antiparkinsonian effects compared with L-dopa.

Other drugs that can be used in Parkinson's disease include **anti-muscarinic drugs** (e.g. trihexyphenidyl [benzhexol], procyclidine) in the early stages where tremor predominates and in some young patients with Parkinson's disease. These drugs are believed to correct a relative overactivity of central cholinergic activation that results from the progressive decrease of (inhibitory) dopaminergic activity. Adverse effects are common and include dry mouth, urinary retention, constipation and confusional states. β-blockers have also been tried for the tremor of Parkinson's disease with some success.

Although most patients with Parkinson's disease are best treated with drugs, surgical approaches have been undertaken in advanced disease. In Parkinson's disease, there is increased activation of the internal part of the globus pallidus and SNr, which in part is mediated by an input from the excitatory subthalamic nucleus. Recent interest has focused on the surgical manipulation of these basal ganglia nuclei, initially in the form of lesions in the GPi (pallidotomy) but more recently with the insertion of electrodes for deep-brain stimulation especially into the subthalamic nucleus. This latter approach may work by generating a temporary lesion, possibly by inducing a conduction block (see Chapters 6 and 8), although this is not proven, and it is now the surgical treatment of choice in advanced Parkinson's disease. This approach seems not only to ameliorate drug-induced problems, but the fundamental motor manifestations of the disease as well. An alternative surgical approach to lesioning or deep-brain stimulation is the implantation of dopamine-rich tissue into the striatum to replace and possibly restore the damaged nigrostriatal pathway. This has been successfully carried out with fetal nigral tissue in a small number of Parkinson's disease patients, although earlier attempts using autografts of the catecholamine-rich adrenal medulla proved unsuccessful. In all cases successful treatment is associated with evidence for a reactivation of the appropriate cortical areas but of late there has been concern about side-effects from this treatment including dyskinesias off therapy post-transplantation—so-called graft-induced dyskinesias. Thus, the use of cell therapies to treat Parkinson's disease is still debatable, as is the use of growth factors such as glial cell line derived neutrotrophic factor (GDNF). In this respect small open label studies have again shown benefit with direct intraputaminal delivery of GDNF into patients with Parkinson's disease, while a more recent double blind placebo controlled trial has not been able to reproduce this.

Huntington's disease

Huntington's disease is an inherited autosomal dominant disorder associated with a trinucleotide expansion in the gene coding for the protein huntingtin on chromosome 4 (see Chapter 60).

The disease presents typically in mid life with a progressive dementia and abnormal movements which usually take the form of chorea—rapid dance-like movements, typically of the hands and neck. This type of movement is described as being hyperkinetic in nature, unlike the hypokinetic deficits seen in Parkinson's disease, and reflects the fact that the primary pathology is the loss of the output neurones of the striatum. This results in relative inhibition of the STN and thus reduced inhibitory outflow from the GPi and SNr, which leads to the cortical motor areas being overactivated, generating an excess of movements.

Treatment of the movement disorder in Huntington's disease is designed to reduce the level of dopaminergic stimulation within the basal ganglia, and is often successful although can cause significant sedation. However, there are no treatments for the cognitive deficits in Huntington's disease, although mood disturbances in this condition often do respond to drugs such as antidepressants (see Chapter 54). As in Parkinson's disease, some progress has been made in the possible use of fetal tissue for transplantation and growth factor (e.g. ciliary neurotrophic factor [CNTF]) delivery to the diseased basal ganglia.

Other disorders of the basal ganglia

Another example of a hyperkinetic movement disorder is *hemiballismus* which is the rapid flailing movements of the limbs contralateral to damage to the subthalamic nucleus.

A number of other conditions can affect the basal ganglia including *Wilson's disease* (an autosomal recessive condition associated with copper deposition); *Sydenham's chorea* (a sequela of rheumatic fever); defects in mitochondrial function (*mitochondrial cytopathies*; see Chapter 60); a number of toxins (e.g. carbon monoxide and manganese); and *choreoathetoid cerebral palsy* (athetosis is defined as an abnormal involuntary slow writhing movement).

The spectrum of movement disorders seen with these diseases is variable because the damage is rarely confined to one structure so patients may exhibit either *parkinsonism, chorea* and *ballismus*, or *dystonia*, where a limb is held in an abnormal fixed posture.

Many of these conditions, including Parkinson's disease and Huntington's disease, have a degree of cognitive impairment—if not frank dementia—and while this may relate to additional damage in the cerebral cortex, there is increasing evidence that it may in part be as a direct result of basal ganglia damage. In this respect the ventral extension of the basal ganglia may be important.

The basal ganglia have a major role in the control of eye movements (see Chapter 42) and so many patients with diseases of the basal ganglia have abnormal eye movements that may be helpful in establishing their clinical diagnosis.

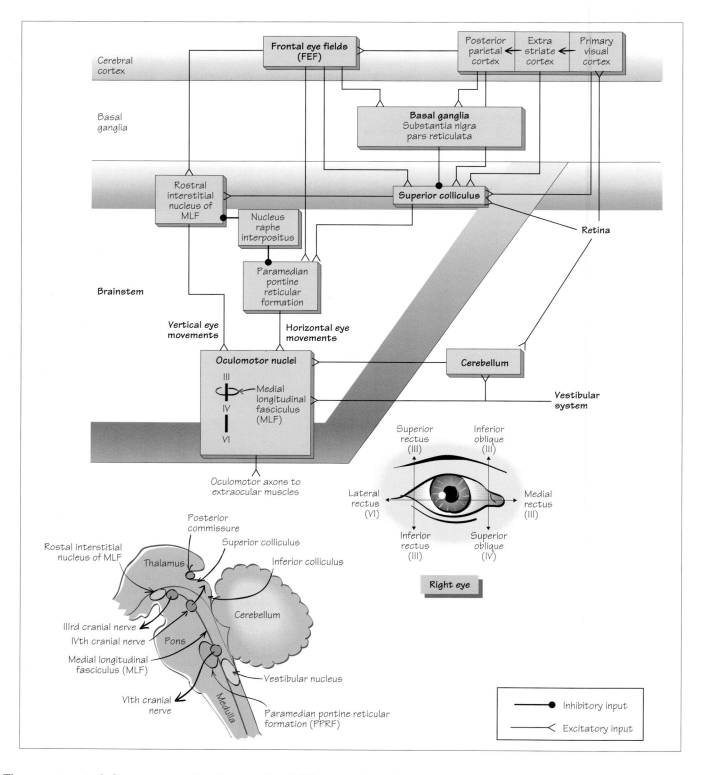

The accurate **control of eye movements** involves a number of different structures, from the extraocular muscles to the frontal cortex, and failure to achieve this control results symptomatically in either double vision (diplopia), blurred vision or oscillopsia (perception of an oscil-

lating image or environmental movement). In clinical practice, disruption of the final pathway from the oculomotor nuclei (third, fourth and sixth cranial nerves) to the extraocular muscle represents one of the major causes of diplopia (e.g. *myasthenia gravis*; see Chapter 7), as does inflammation (e.g. *multiple sclerosis*) in the medial longitudinal fasciculus (MLF) pathway linking the oculomotor nuclei.

Types of eye movement

There are three major types of eye movement.

1 Smooth pursuit or the following of a target accurately, which is controlled primarily by posterior parts of the cortex in conjunction with the cerebellum.

2 Saccadic eye movements where there is a sudden shift of the eyes to a new target and which are controlled by more anterior cortical areas, the basal ganglia and superior colliculus in the midbrain.

3 Sustained gaze where the eyes are fixed in one direction and which is primarily a function of the brainstem (especially the paramedian pontine reticular formation [PPRF] and rostral interstitial nucleus of the MLF).

Eye movements, like the motor system in general, can be either **voluntary** (when the command comes from the frontal eye field) or **reflex** (when the command originates from subcortical structures and posterior parietal cortex).

Manifestations of disordered eye movement include a loss of conjugate movements; broken pursuit movements; inaccurate saccades; gaze palsies; and nystagmus. **Nystagmus** is defined as a biphasic ocular oscillation containing an abnormal slow and corrective fast phase, the latter defining the direction of the nystagmus.

Anatomy and physiology of central nervous system control of eye movements

• The **frontal eye fields** (FEF; predominantly Brodmann's area 8) are found anterior to the premotor cortex (PMC; see Chapter 37). Stimulation of this structure produces eye movements, typically saccades, to the contralateral side, and may be seen clinically in some epileptic patients.

Damage to this area reduces the ability to look to the contralateral side so the patient tends to look towards the side of the lesion. The FEF primarily receives from the posterior parietal cortex and projects to the superior colliculus, other brainstem centres and the basal ganglia.

• The **posterior parietal cortex** (corresponds to Brodmann's area 7 in monkeys) contains a large number of neurones responsive to complex visual stimuli, as well as coding for some visually guided eye movements (see Chapter 32). It is especially important in the generation of saccades to objects of visual significance via its connections with the FEF and superior colliculus.

Damage to this area, in addition to causing deficiencies in visual attention and saccades to objects in the contralateral hemifield, can impair smooth pursuit eye movements as evidenced by loss of the **optokinetic reflex**. This is a reflex in which the eyes fixate by a series of rapid movements on a moving target, such as a rotating drum, with vertical lines as fixation targets.

• The **primary visual cortex and its associated extrastriate areas** are involved in both saccadic and smooth pursuit eye movements (see Chapters 26 and 27). Their role in saccadic movements is primarily through the projection of V1 to the superior colliculus, while the role in smooth pursuit is via extrastriate area V5 (see Chapter 27), and projections to the FEF, posterior parietal cortex and pons.

Damage to the striate and extrastriate areas, in addition to producing field defects and specific deficiencies of visual function (see Chapter 27), can also cause major abnormalities in smooth pursuit eye movements.

• The **basal ganglia** have a major role in the control of saccadic eye movements (see Chapters 40 and 41). The caudate nucleus receives from the FEF and projects via the substantia nigra pars reticulata to the superior colliculus.

Abnormalities in saccadic eye movements are seen clinically in a number of basal ganglia disorders. For example, in *Parkinson's disease* the saccadic eye movements tend to be slightly inaccurate with undershooting to the target (hypometric saccades).

• The **superior colliculus** in the midbrain is important in the accurate execution of saccades (see Chapter 26).

• The **cerebellum and vestibular nuclei** have important complex inputs into the brainstem oculomotor system and are especially important in the control of pursuit movements, as well as mediating the vestibulo-ocular reflex (see Chapters 30, 39 and 50).

Damage to the cerebellum and vestibular system causes broken pursuit eye movements, inaccurate saccades and nystagmus.

• The **rostral interstitial nucleus of the medial longitudinal fasciculus (riMLF)** is important in the control of vertical saccades and vertical gaze (both up- and downgaze) and receives important inputs from the FEF and superior colliculus while projecting to all the oculomotor nuclei.

Damage to this structure or disruption of its afferent inputs therefore produces deficiencies in both these eye movements, and this can occur in a number of conditions including some neurodegenerative diseases.

• The **PPRF** receives from the FEF, superior colliculus and cerebellum and is responsible for horizontal saccades and gaze. It is thought that this structure may work in conjunction with another pontine nucleus, the **nucleus raphe interpositus**. This latter nucleus contains omnipause neurones, which normally exert tonic inhibition on the burst neurones of the PPRF (and riMLF) mediating the saccadic impulse.

Damage to nucleus raphe interpositus results in random chaotic eye movements or *opsoclonus*. In contrast, damage to the PPRF causes deficiencies in saccadic eye movements as well as ipsilateral gaze paresis.

• The **MLF** mediates conjugate eye movements through interconnections between all the oculomotor nuclei and is commonly affected in some diseases of the CNS, such as *multiple sclerosis* (see Chapter 59).

A lesion in this structure causes an *internuclear ophthalmoplegia*, with nystagmus in the abducting eye and slowed or absent adduction in the other eye.

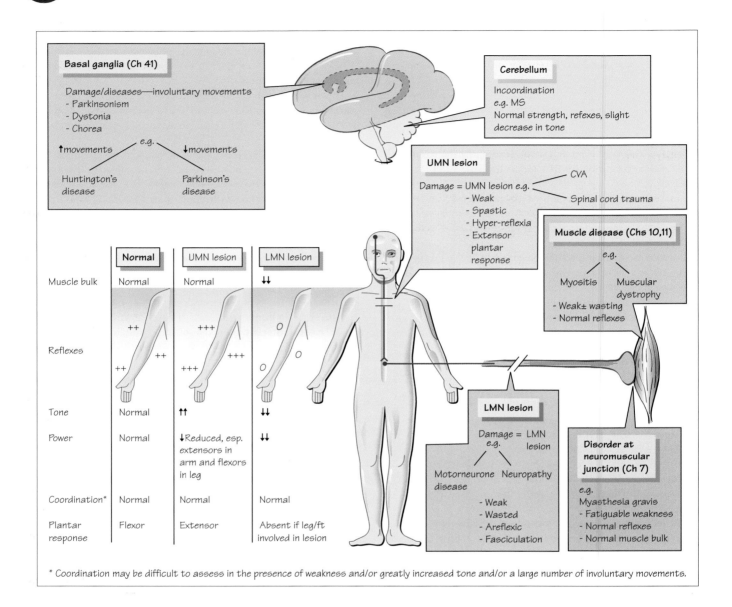

Basal ganglia (Ch 41)

Damage/diseases—involuntary movements
- Parkinsonism
- Dystonia
- Chorea

↑movements — e.g. — ↓movements

Huntington's disease / Parkinson's disease

Cerebellum

Incoordination
e.g. MS
Normal strength, refexes, slight decrease in tone

UMN lesion

Damage = UMN lesion e.g. — CVA
- Weak — Spinal cord trauma
- Spastic
- Hyper-reflexia
- Extensor plantar response

Muscle disease (Chs 10,11)

e.g.

Myositis / Muscular dystrophy

- Weak± wasting
- Normal reflexes

	Normal	UMN lesion	LMN lesion
Muscle bulk	Normal	Normal	↓↓
Reflexes	++ ++ ++	+++ +++ +++	0 0 0
Tone	Normal	↑↑	↓↓
Power	Normal	↓Reduced, esp. extensors in arm and flexors in leg	↓↓
Coordination*	Normal	Normal	Normal
Plantar response	Flexor	Extensor	Absent if leg/ft involved in lesion

LMN lesion

Damage = LMN lesion e.g.

Motorneurone disease / Neuropathy

- Weak
- Wasted
- Areflexic
- Fasciculation

Disorder at neuromuscular junction (Ch 7)

e.g.
Myasthesia gravis
- Fatiguable weakness
- Normal reflexes
- Normal muscle bulk

*Coordination may be difficult to assess in the presence of weakness and/or greatly increased tone and/or a large number of involuntary movements.

Disturbances in the motor pathways can produce a range of disorders of movement. These typically involve the muscle, causing weakness; the neuromuscular junction (NMJ), causing fatiguable weakness; the motorneurones (lower or upper), giving weakness and changes in muscle tone and reflexes; the cerebellum and its connections, causing problems with coordination without any changes in power or reflexes; and the basal ganglia, which produces an abnormal involuntary movement without any effect on power, reflexes or coordination.

In order to determine the nature and cause of the motor disturbance a full history and examination are needed along with appropriate tests. The majority of patients with isolated motor symptoms have either Parkinson's or motorneurone disease, although by far the most common clinical scenario is the patient with both motor and sensory abnormalities as a result of strokes or damaged nerves as they emerge or pass along the limb.

A typical screen of tests for patients with motor symptoms involves blood tests, nerve conduction studies (NCS), electromyography (EMG) and magnetic resonance imaging (MRI) of brain and spinal cord.

Muscle (see Chapters 10 and 11)

The typical features of a muscle disease are weakness, which may relate to exercise, and on occasions muscle pain (myalgia). The age and rate of progression is often helpful in determining the type of muscle disease, e.g. progressive slow weakness without pain from childhood would suggest a degenerative *muscular dystrophy* (see Chapter 10) while a short history of painful weakness in adulthood would suggest an *inflammatory myositis* (see Chapter 59). The distribution of weakness is also helpful in defining the likely type of muscle disease, e.g. proximal arm and leg weakness in *limb girdle muscular dystrophy*. The investigations that are especially useful in muscle disease are blood tests to look at levels of muscle-specific creatine phosphokinase (CPK)—a measure of muscle damage; EMG and muscle biopsy. In some cases genetic testing is of value, especially if the muscle weakness is associated with myotonia and the other features of *myotonic dystrophy*.

Neuromuscular junction (see Chapter 7 and 59)

Patients with these disorders present with a history of weakness that gets worse with continued use of the muscle. The most common disorder of the NMJ is *myasthenia gravis*, which typically presents in early or late adulthood with fatiguable diplopia, ptosis, facial and bulbar weakness and proximal limb weakness. The examination confirms weakness that may be present at rest but clearly gets worse with exercise. Patients can present as a neurological emergency if there is bulbar and respiratory failure. Diagnosis typically relies on history and examination, the presence of acetylcholine receptor (AChR) or muscle-specific kinase (MUSK) antibodies, a positive response to a short-acting acetylcholinesterase inhibitor (Tensilon test) and abnormalities on repetitive stimulation with NCS and EMG. Muscle biopsy is not necessary. In some patients myasthenia gravis is associated with either enlargement (hyperplasia) or a tumour of the thymus gland. Other myasthenic syndromes are rare.

Peripheral nerve

Damage to the peripheral nerves will generally give both sensory and motor symptoms and signs. However, the peripheral motor nerve can be preferentially involved in some neuropathies as well as in conditions such as *poliomyelitis* and *motorneurone disease*, which target the actual motorneurone cell body in the ventral horn of the spinal cord and/or brainstem. The typical features of damage to the peripheral motor nerve are weakness, wasting, fasciculation and loss of reflexes—a lower motorneurone (LMN) lesion. Investigation of LMN syndromes involves excluding nerve entrapment as it comes out of the spinal cord by MRI imaging, along with NCS and EMG—the latter showing features of denervation with spontaneous motor discharges from the muscle that has lost its normal innervation.

Spinal cord

The involvement of spinal cord pathways gives a variety of motor syndromes (see Chapters 34 and 36). In rare cases there is involvement of spinal cord interneurones giving continuous motor unit activity (CMUA) and a *stiff-man syndrome* (see Chapter 36). Involvement of descending motor pathways from the brain in the spinal cord gives an upper motorneurone (UMN) syndrome of weakness, spasticity, increased reflexes, and clonus and extensor plantars. It is unusual for this pathway to be selectively involved in spinal cord pathology and when it is the patient often also has LMN signs and has a form of motorneurone disease called *amyotrophic lateral sclerosis or Lou Gehrig disease*. However, if only UMN signs are seen then the patient is said to have *primary lateral sclerosis*. Structural lesions of the spinal cord typically produce a combination of motor and sensory signs and symptoms. Investigation involves MRI, with cerebrospinal fluid (CSF) examination if an inflammatory aetiology is suspected and in some cases neurophysiological testing with EMG, NCS and central motor conduction time (CMCT).

Brain

Damage to supraspinal structures can produce a variety of motor signs and symptoms. Involvement is most commonly seen in *cerebrovascular accidents (CVAs)* with involvement of all the descending motor pathways from the cortex to the brainstem and spinal cord. This gives rise to a contralateral hemiparesis with UMN signs. If the left hemisphere is involved there is typically a major disturbance in speech. Occasionally, damage is restricted to the motor cortex, when the patient may present with focal motor seizures such as *Jacksonian epilepsy* (see Chapters 37 and 38). The mainstay of investigation of supraspinal motor abnormalities is MRI and/or computerized tomography (CT) imaging and CSF examination if an inflammatory aetiology is suspected. In some cases genetic testing is helpful.

Other sites commonly involved in disease processes

Basal ganglia

Produces either a slowness of movement such as in *Parkinson's disease*; an abnormality of limb posture and movement (*dystonia*) or the development of uncontrollable involuntary movements such as *chorea* and *hemiballismus* (see Chapter 41).

Cerebellum

Produces incoordination of movement with slurred speech and abnormal eye movements (see Chapter 39). The disease processes that typically affect this part of the CNS are *multiple sclerosis*, drugs such as anticonvulsants and alcohol along with a series of rare genetic conditions called the *spinocerebellar ataxias (SCAs)* (see Chapter 60). It can also be involved by tumour growth in which case the situation may be complicated by the development of *hydrocephalus* through compression of the fourth ventricle and its outflow foramina (see Chapter 18).

44

The reticular formation and sleep

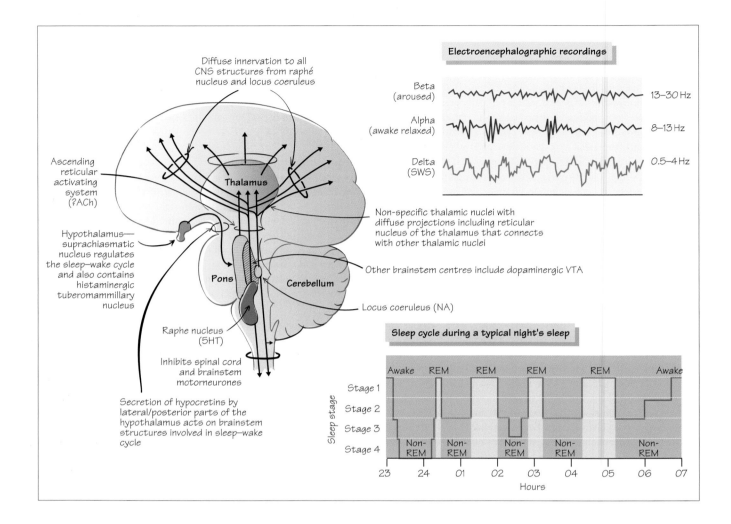

Sleep

Sleep is a characteristic of all mammals and is defined behaviourally as a reduced responsiveness to environmental stimuli, and electrophysiologically by specific changes in electroencephalographic (EEG) activity. In addition, there are a number of changes associated with autonomic nervous system (ANS) function.

Normal patterns of sleep are essential for human well-being, although it is still unclear why we need to dream.

EEG patterns during states of consciousness and slow-wave sleep

EEG recordings from normal awake subjects at rest show a characteristic high-frequency (13–30 Hz, β **activity**) low-voltage pattern. This desynchronized activity changes as the subject closes his or her eyes and becomes drowsy, with the new EEG pattern having a lower frequency (8–13 Hz, α **activity**) but slightly higher voltage. This pattern is said to be synchronized and results from the simultaneous firing of many cortical neurones following thalamocortical activity.

EEG studies have revealed that sleep occurs in characteristic stages. As the subject falls asleep (stage 1), the EEG is similar to the awake EEG (low-voltage, fast activity). As sleep deepens through stages 2 and 3 to stage 4, the EEG amplitude progressively increases and its frequency falls. Stage 3 and 4 sleep is called collectively slow-wave sleep (SWS) or **non-rapid eye movement** (non-REM) sleep because the eyes are still. After about 90 min of sleep, the EEG changes back to a low-voltage, fast pattern that is indistinguishable from stage 1 non-REM sleep. However, during this phase of sleep there are rapid eye movements. This type of sleep is called **rapid eye movement sleep** (REM sleep), or paradoxical sleep because although the EEG is similar to that of an awake person, sleepers are difficult to arouse and muscle tone is absent. Most dreaming occurs during REM sleep although that occurring during non-REM sleep is said to be have a higher emotional content with less detail.

Neural mechanisms of sleep

In contrast to the popular notion of 'falling' asleep, sleep is an active process involving a number of neurotransmitter systems. Levels of consciousness reflect a balance between systems promoting arousal and sleep. Cholinergic neurones in the **ascending reticular activating system** projects via two pathways: a dorsal route via the medial thalamus and the ventral path via the lateral hypothalamus, basal ganglia and forebrain. Extensive thalamocortical projections provide the basis for widespread changes in cortical cell excitability. Activity in cholinergic neurones lead to an increase in arousal and cortical desynchrony. Activity in this system is also responsible for the pontine–geniculo-occipital (PGO) waves, an indicator of the onset of REM sleep. Our understanding of the role of monoamines in sleep processes is incomplete. Both noradrenergic neurones in the locus coeruleus and serotoninergic (5-hydroxytryptamine [5-HT]) neurones in the raphe nuclei are involved in controlling the balance between different sleep stages and sleep and arousal. Neurones in the ventrolateral preoptic area (VLPA) send an inhibitory γ-aminobutyric acid (GABA)-mediated input to the locus coeruleus, raphe nuclei and tuberomammilary nucleus. The latter contains histaminergic neurones which are likely to be the substrate for the sedative effects of antihistamine drugs. Other brain regions implicated in sleep and arousal patterns include the suprachiasmatic nucleus of the hypothalamus. Clearly, drugs such as alcohol, benzodiazepines, antidepressants and the antihistamines all have significant influences on these transmitter systems.

More recently, a number of peptides have been identified as being associated with sleep states (e.g. Orexins and delta sleep-inducing peptide [DSIP]). It is unclear what relationship these peptides have with the neural mechanisms described above. However, because Siamese twins have different sleep patterns but a shared circulation it seems unlikely that chemical mediators of sleep have a very significant role.

Sleep disorders

Insomnia is the most common sleep disorder. It can be defined as the failure to obtain the required amount or quality of sleep to function normally during the day. *Primary insomnia* supposedly brought about by dysfunction of sleep mechanisms in the brain is rare, but these patients are the ones who may require treatment with hypnotic drugs. Causes of secondary insomnia include psychiatric disease (especially depression and anxiety disorders), physical disorders, chronic pain, drug misuse (e.g. excessive alcohol, caffeine), personal crises and old age.

Management of insomnia

Hypnotics are drugs that promote sleep. They include drugs acting at the benzodiazepine receptor (benzodiazepines and Z-drugs), chloral hydrate, chlormethiazole and barbiturates. **Benzodiazepines** and the more recent **Z-drugs** are by far the most widely used hypnotics. They also have anxiolytic, anticonvulsant, muscle relaxant and amnesic actions. All the actions of benzodiazepines are believed to be caused by the enhancement of GABA-mediated inhibition in the central nervous system (CNS). $GABA_A$ receptors possess several 'modulatory' sites including one for benzodiazepines, which when activated causes a conformational change in the GABA receptor. This increases the affinity of GABA binding and enhances the actions of GABA on the Cl^- conductance of the neuronal membrane.

Any benzodiazepine given at night will induce sleep but a rapidly eliminated drug (e.g. **temazepam**) is usually preferred to avoid daytime sedation. Some newer drugs do not have the benzodiazepine structure but are benzodiazepine-receptor agonists. These are the so-called Z-drugs, **zopiclone, zolpidem and zaleplon**. Mouse mutation studies in which the α_1-subunit of the benzodiazepine receptor is inactivated, have revealed that zolpidem and zaleplon become inactive, indicating a selective action on the α_1-subtype (see also Chapter 56). The Z-drugs have shorter half-lives than the benzodiazepines and are less likely to cause daytime sedation. Also they have a reduced propensity to tolerance and withdrawal and less abuse liability. For these reasons they are increasingly popular for the management of insomnia.

The benzodiazepines are central depressants but their maximum effect when given orally does not normally cause fatal respiratory depression (in contrast to opioids or barbiturates). Adverse effects include drowsiness, impaired alertness and ataxia as well as a low-grade dependence after a few weeks' use. Withdrawal of the drug may cause a physical withdrawal syndrome (anxiety, insomnia) that may last for weeks.

For many cases of insomnia, psychological strategies may be effective alternatives to drugs.

Hypersomnia (daytime sleepiness)

This is a serious but less common complaint than insomnia. Common causes of persistent daytime sleepiness include narcolepsy, obstructive sleep apnoea, drugs (e.g. benzodiazepines, alcohol) and depression (20% have hypersomnia rather than insomnia).

Narcolepsy

Narcolepsy is characterized by irresistable sleep episodes lasting 5–30 min during the day often in association with cataplexy (loss of muscle tone and temporary paralysis) usually provoked by emotion, e.g. laughter, anger, as well as sleep paralysis and hallucinations at the time of going to or waking up from sleep. It has a very strong histocompatibility locus antigen (HLA) association (DR2/DQW1) and, while no pathological abnormalities have been detected in these patients, it is probable that there are abnormalities in the brainstem structures underlying sleep, as there is evidence of short latency REM sleep during normal waking hours. In addition, the identification of the novel neuropeptides **hypocretins or orexins** may be important, as these substances are synthesized in the hypothalamus and act on a number of brainstem centres important in the regulation of sleep. Indeed, deficiencies in these peptides have recently been described in narcolepsy in some patients and a number of animal models. The syndrome has a devastating effect on quality of life, which may be improved by long-term treatment with stimulants, e.g. dexamfetamine, methylphenidate and modafinil. Clomipramine is used to treat the cataplexy.

Obstructive sleep apnoea syndrome

This occurs if the upper airway at the back of the throat collapses when the patient breathes during sleep. This reduces the oxygen in the blood, which arouses the patient causing him or her to momentarily awake and prevents a normal sleep pattern. The patient, usually an overweight man, is often unaware of these awakenings, but the disruption to sleep results in daytime sleepiness and impaired daytime performance. It can be treated by weight loss, positive ventilatory support at night and, occasionally, oropharyngeal surgery. If it is not treated it can lead to long-term cardiorespiratory problems such as pulmonary hypertension and right heart failure.

45

Consciouness, theory of mind and general anaesthesia

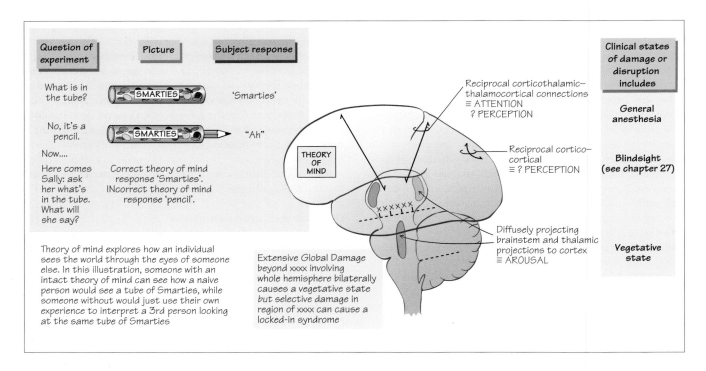

In this chapter we discuss what is meant by consciousness, and how this can be altered in certain pathological conditions as well as pharmacologically by general anaesthesia (see also Chapter 44). This ability to be aware of what we are doing, namely consciousness, is then discussed further in terms of how we can understand the thought processes of others, so-called theory of mind, disorders of which may underlie a range of conditions especially *autism*.

Consciousness—what is it?

In thinking about consciousness, it is important to differentiate between the **level** and the **content** of conscious experience. **The level of consciousness** may also be referred to as the level of **arousal** while the **contents of consciousness** refers to the objects and occurrences of which we are aware. Of course, the contents of consciousness will be affected greatly by the level of consciousness but these two phenomena are likely to be at least partly dissociable. For example, people in hyperaroused states may be less aware of surroundings than less aroused individuals. Conversely, it has recently been shown that individuals in a **vegetative state** may actually show neurophysiological patterns of activity (as measured by functional magnetic resonance imaging [fMRI]; see Chapter 53) that indicates a much richer level of awareness than their immobile unresponsive state would suggest.

In general, experimental and clinical access to the contents of consciousness relies upon verbal report and certain behavioural indicators. We may ask a subject to tell us or to indicate whether they are aware of a stimulus in the periphery of their visual field. We may assess their memory by requiring them to indicate whether they have an awareness of whether a particular stimulus was previously presented to them. We may also attempt to measure the richness of their awareness through such measures; with respect to memory, for example, does the

subject truly recollect a prior presentation or do they simply have a strong sense that it is familiar?

An important observation with respect to the contents of consciousness is that while our awareness obviously defines our experience of the world, the explanations that they provide for our behaviour is only partial and may be inaccurate. This was shown strikingly in an experiment by Libet and colleagues who required volunteers to make periodic movements while simultaneously recording cerebral activity. They showed that subjective assessments of becoming aware of an intention to move actually occurred some 500 ms after there had been a brain response. This finding, subsequently replicated, suggests that our brain can indicate what we are about to do before we ourselves are aware of wanting to do it. Further evidence of a discrepancy between what we are aware of and what we actually do comes from work by Castiello and colleagues who showed that when subjects receive incorrect feedback about the trajectory of an arm movement that they are in the process of making, they will correct the movement without actually being aware of doing so, even when the correction made is relatively large. Furthermore, when asked to reproduce the movement that they have just made, subjects will reproduce the one that mirrors the incorrect feedback that they were given, further suggesting that they were unconscious of the control that they have exerted over the movement.

It is also the case that previously experienced events or objects may influence our ongoing actions and decisions without necessarily re-emerging into consciousness. The occurrence of basic processing outside our awareness would seem to be an efficient way of freeing our conscious processing to deal with more complex problems. However, it should be remembered that there are clear instances where the contents of consciousness may have a marked impact upon lower-level processes. For example, Haggard and colleagues showed that subjects who have made a willed (conscious) movement are likely to link more closely in time that movement with an outcome than when the movement is not felt to be consciously initiated (if it is produced by application of a brief magnetic field over the motor cortex). Thus, consciousness enables actions to gain greater prominence in our memory, but much of what we do routinely does not require this to happen. As to the precise neurobiological origin of consciousness, this is unknown, but the coordinated activity of the cortex and its reciprocal connections to the thalamus and diffusely projecting brainstem nuclei are important. This is best illustrated in patients in a *vegetative state* (see below) and *blindsight* (see Chapter 27). In this latter condition there is damage to the primary visual cortex such that individuals cannot consciously see but when tested it is clear that their visual system can detect visual stimuli of different forms including colour and motion. This is thought to arise from the intact extrastriate visual areas, which cannot feedback to the primary visual cortex and as a result conscious visual perception is lost.

Consciousness and theory of mind

As humans, we may be unique in being conscious of our consciouness. This thinking about thinking has been referred to as 'meta-representation' and it is perhaps the ability to represent our own mental states and those of others that facilitates and shapes our most complex social interactions. To be able to represent the mental states of others has been referred to as having a '**theory of mind**'. We must use this theory of mind to interpret, explain and predict many of the actions and utterances of other people. If someone is being sarcastic or deceitful, they say and do precisely the opposite of what they feel. By understanding these possibilities their behaviour may become more logical and predictable to us.

What happens if we have difficulty with theory of mind processing? It has been suggested that the isolation and very limited social repertoire of individuals with *autism* may arise from the difficulty that they have in understanding the mental states of other people. There is also evidence that people with *schizophrenia* may have deficits in theory of mind abilities and in both cases the abnormality underlying this deficit is thought to reside in the prefrontal cortex (see Chapter 55).

Vegetative state

Some patients who have a major global brain injury (e.g. anoxia secondary to a cardiac or respiratory arrest) can end up in a state of unresponsive wakefulness or a *vegetative state* (which is said to be permenant if it continues for more than six months to a year depending on the nature of the original insult). In this state the patient clearly has periods of sleep and wakefulness, but during the latter time they are unable to respond to any stimuli as there is extensive damage above the level of the arousal systems in the brainstem. In some cases the responses to such stimuli are present, but inconsistently so, and such individuals are deemed to be in a *minimally conscious state (MCS)*. However, it is important that all individuals in a vegetative state or MCS are investigated thoroughly over time using a range of stimuli and functional imaging (see Chapter 53), as some patients appear not to be able to respond, while nevertheless showing evidence for cortical activation with sensory stimuli on functional imaging. In these cases the patient may have had a more focal injury to the upper brainstem that prevents them from being able to make any clear motor responses to stimuli—the so-called *locked in syndrome*. Once recognized, such patients may be able to communicate through the use of eye movements and blinking (see Chapter 42).

General anaesthesia

The ability to switch off consciousness using drugs is routinely performed in medical practice through the use of general anaesthetics, which are administered to patients undergoing surgical procedures as well as patients with major medical problems on intensive care units. These agents are given by intravenous injection or by inhalation and act to switch off the diffusely projecting brainstem and thalamocortical networks, which are thought to mediate arousal and consciouness.

Understanding of how general anaesthetics produce loss of consciousness is poor for most agents. A striking feature of anaesthetics is the huge range of chemical structures that can produce anaesthesia. These vary from the element xenon, through simple organic chemicals such as ether to the more complex steroid anaesthetics.

An early finding was that the oil–water partition coefficients of these diverse chemicals correlated extremely well with their anaesthetic potency. This led to the '**lipid' theory** of anaesthesia, the idea being that the anaesthetic dissolved in the lipid bilayers of the nerve membrane causing expansion and increased fluidity. The resulting disorder in the membrane may alter ionic fluxes (see Chapter 6) and produce anaesthesia. This simple idea that anaesthetics act '**non-specifically**' could account for the chemical diversity of anaesthetics, but it is now generally accepted that they act by binding to hydrophobic regions of sensitive target proteins, e.g. ion channels. In the case of some intravenous agents, e.g. propofol, there is strong evidence that they bind to the $GABA_A$ receptor and by enhancing GABAergic transmission, produce anaesthesia (cf. benzodiazepines; see Chapter 44).The molecular targets for inhalational agents are less clear. Some, e.g. halothane, isoflurane, servoflurane, enhance GABAergic transmission, but others, e.g. nitrous oxide, do not. All volatile anaesthetics potentiate the action of glycine receptors and some potassium channels are activated by anaesthetics. The latter effects are usually small but may cause a substantial decrease in neuronal excitability.

Intravenous agents

These drugs cause rapid loss of consciousness. They may be used alone for minor procedures but are used mainly for the induction of anaesthesia. **Thiopental**, a highly lipid-soluble barbiturate, produces anaesthesia in less than 30 s. This drug was used widely but has largely been replaced by **propofol**, an agent that causes less myocardial depression and is associated with rapid recovery without nausea or hangover.

Inhalation agents

Nitrous oxide at concentrations up to 70% is the most widely used anaesthetic agent. It is used as a carrier gas for volatile agents. It produces sedation and analgesia but is not sufficient alone to maintain anaesthesia. Nitrous oxide has little effect on the cardiovascular or respiratory systems.

Halothane was the first fluorinated anaesthetic. Its vapour is non-irritant and induction is smooth and pleasant. Halothane causes hypotension by depressing the myocardium. More importantly, it often sensitizes the heart to catecholamines and often causes arrhythmias. Metabolites of halothane may cause severe hepatotoxicity and for this reason halothane has been replaced by newer, less toxic drugs.

Isoflurane, desflurane and sevoflurane do not sensitize the heart to epinephrine and, because only a tiny proportion of the administered dose is metabolized, are unlikely to be hepatotoxic.

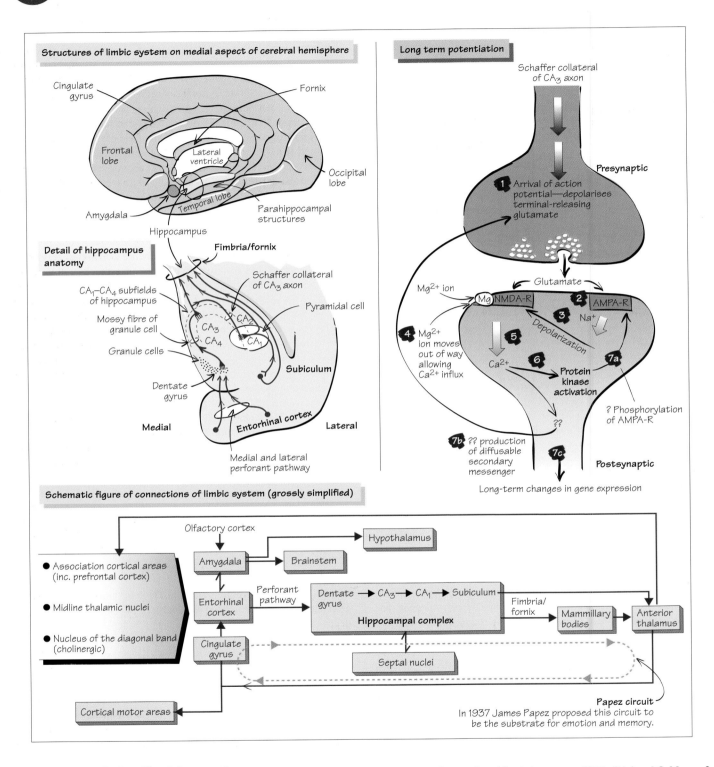

Structures of limbic system on medial aspect of cerebral hemisphere

Cingulate gyrus
Fornix
Frontal lobe
Lateral ventricle
Occipital lobe
Amygdala
Temporal lobe
Parahippocampal structures
Hippocampus

Detail of hippocampus anatomy

Fimbria/fornix
CA_1–CA_4 subfields of hippocampus
Schaffer collateral of CA_3 axon
Pyramidal cell
Mossy fibre of granule cell
CA_3
CA_2
CA_4
CA_1
Granule cells
Subiculum
Dentate gyrus
Medial
Entorhinal cortex
Lateral
Medial and lateral perforant pathway

Long term potentiation

Schaffer collateral of CA_3 axon
Presynaptic
1 Arrival of action potential—depolarises terminal-releasing glutamate
Glutamate
Mg^{2+} ion
Mg NMDA-R
2 AMPA-R
3 Na^+
Depolarization
4 Mg^{2+} ion moves out of way allowing Ca^{2+} influx
5
Ca^{2+}
6
Protein kinase activation
7a
? Phosphorylation of AMPA-R
??
7b ?? production of diffusable secondary messenger
7c
Postsynaptic
Long-term changes in gene expression

Schematic figure of connections of limbic system (grossly simplified)

Olfactory cortex
Hypothalamus
● Association cortical areas (inc. prefrontal cortex)
Amygdala
Brainstem
● Midline thalamic nuclei
Entorhinal cortex
Perforant pathway
Dentate gyrus → CA_3 → CA_1 → Subiculum
Fimbria/fornix
Mammillary bodies
Anterior thalamus
● Nucleus of the diagonal band (cholinergic)
Hippocampal complex
Cingulate gyrus
Septal nuclei
Cortical motor areas
Papez circuit
In 1937 James Papez proposed this circuit to be the substrate for emotion and memory.

Anatomy of the limbic system

The **limbic system** refers to a collection of areas that lie primarily along the medial aspect of the temporal lobe and includes the **cingulate gyrus**, **parahippocampal structures (postsubiculum, parasubiculum, presubiculum and perirhinal cortex)**, **entorhinal cortex**, **hippocampal complex (dentate gyrus, CA1–CA4 subfields and subiculum), septal nuclei and amygdala**. Additional structures closely associated with it include the mammillary bodies of the hypothalamus, olfactory cortex and nucleus accumbens (see Chapters 17, 31, 40 and 48, respectively).

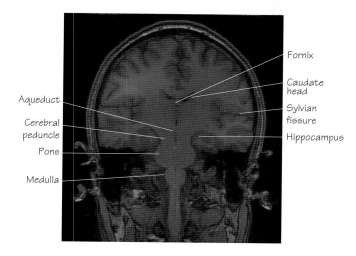

Aqueduct
Cerebral peduncle
Pons
Medulla

Fornix
Caudate head
Sylvian fissure
Hippocampus

recognize facial expressions of fear. Conversely, stimulation of this structure produces a pattern of behaviour typical of fear with increased autonomic activity. This is sometimes seen clinically in **temporal lobe epilepsy** where patients complain of brief episodes of fear.

Cingulate gyrus

The cingulate gyrus running around the medial aspect of the whole hemisphere has a number of functions, including a role in complex motor control (see Chapter 37), pain perception (see Chapters 23 and 24) and social interactions.

Damage to this structure can produce motor neglect, as well as reduced pain perception, reduced aggressiveness and vocalization, emotional blunting and altered social behaviour which can result in a clinical state of **akinetic mutism** (not talking or moving). Stimulation of this area, either experimentally or during an epileptic seizure, produces alterations in the autonomic outflow and motor arrest, with vocalization and complex movements.

Long-term potentiation

Long-term potentiation (LTP) is defined as an increase in the strength of synaptic transmission with repetitive use that lasts for more than a few minutes, and in the hippocampus it can be triggered by less than 1 s of intense synaptic activity and lasts for hours or much longer. It can be induced at a number of central nervous system (CNS) sites but especially the hippocampus and it has therefore been postulated to be important in **memory acquisition**. However, different mechanisms may underlie LTP at different synapses within the hippocampal complex, and that most of the work is based on the excitatory glutamate synapse in the CA1 subfield of the hippocampal complex.

The current model of LTP is as follows.
- An afferent burst of activity leads to the release of glutamate from the presynaptic terminal (stage 1 on figure).
- The released glutamate then binds to both NMDA and non-NMDA receptors in the postsynaptic membrane. These latter receptors lead to a Na^+ influx (stage 2) which depolarizes the postsynaptic membrane (stage 3).
- The depolarization of the postsynaptic membrane not only leads to an excitatory postsynaptic potential (EPSP), but also removes Mg^{2+} from the NMDA-associated ion channel (stage 4). The Mg^{2+} normally blocks the NMDA-R associated ion channel and thus its removal in response to postsynaptic depolarization allows a further Na^+ and Ca^{2+} influx into the postsynaptic cell (stage 5).
- The Ca^{2+} influx leads to the activation of a postsynaptic protein kinase (stage 6), which is responsible for the initial **induction of LTP**—a postsynaptic event.
- The **maintenance of LTP**, in addition to requiring a persistent activation of protein kinase activity (stage 7a), the insertion possibly of more postsynaptic glutamate receptors and changes in gene transcription (stage 7c), may also require a modification of neurotransmitter release (stage 7b), i.e. an increase in transmitter release in response to a given afferent impulse. The presynaptic modification, if necessary in the maintenance of LTP, means that the postsynaptic cell must produce a diffusible secondary signal that can act on the presynaptic terminal such as permeant arachidonic acid metabolites, nitric oxide, carbon monoxide and platelet activating factor.

In some circumstances **long-term depression (LTD)** can be induced in the mossy fibre synapses in the CA3 subfield of the hippocampus. This, in contrast to LTP, is thought to be mediated by a presynaptic metabotropic glutamate receptor.

The **anatomical organization** of the limbic system indicates that it performs some high-level processing of sensory information, given its input from the association cortices (see Chapter 32). The predominant outflow of the limbic system is to the prefrontal cortex and hypothalamus as well as to cortical areas involved with the planning of behaviour, including motor response (see Chapters 34 and 37). Thus, anatomically the limbic system appears to have a role in attaching a behavioural significance and response to a stimulus, especially with respect to its emotional content. The hippocampal complex has been shown to have both a high degree of susceptibility to hypoxia and yet a remarkable degree of plasticity which helps explain why this structure is important in the generation of epileptic seizures (see Chapter 58) as well as memory acquisition. It is also one of the major sites for neurogenesis in the adult brain, which may also be important in this mnemonic and mood functions.

Function of the limbic system

Hippocampal complex and parahippocampal structures

(see also Chapter 47)

The original description in the 1950s by Scoville and Milner of patient H.M. with bilateral anterior temporal lobectomy and a resulting profound amnesic state suggested that this area of the brain had a major role in memory. Subsequently, the hippocampus proper and parahippocampal areas have a role in the ability to acquire information about events (see Chapter 47), although the major role of the hippocampus itself probably relates more to spatial memory.

However, the long-term storage of memories occurs at a site distant and is probably within the overlying cerebral cortex—as demonstrated by the pattern of memory loss seen in **dementia of the Alzheimer type** (DAT; see Chapter 57), namely well-preserved retrograde memory (for distant events such as childhood) in the face of severely impaired or absent anterograde memory (inability to remember what the patient has just done).

Amygdala (see also Chapter 48)

The amygdala is a small almond-shaped structure made up of many nuclei that lies on the medial aspect of the temporal lobe.

Damage to this structure experimentally leads to blunted emotional reactions to normally arousing stimuli, and can even prevent the acquisition of emotional behaviour. In humans with selective amygdala damage there appears to be a profound impairment in the ability to

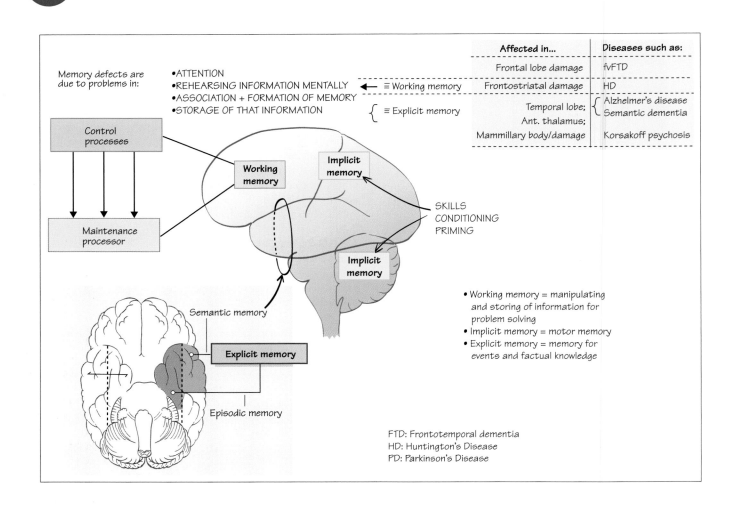

The term memory is commonly used to refer to the ability to remember information but it is important to understand that there are several **different types of memory** that subserve different functions. In the first instance there is a distinction between motor and non-motor memories—the former is a form of **implicit memory** and typically involves the cerebellum, motor cortical areas and basal ganglia (see Chapters 37–41) and will not be discussed further in this chapter. The other forms of memory are more involved with the taking in, manipulating and storing of information for problem solving (**working memory**), events and factual knowledge (**explicit memory**).

In clinical practice it is not uncommon for patients and their families to complain about disorders of memory when they are referring to a range of different cognitive problems such as a deficit in language (see Chapter 29), attention or perception (see Chapter 32). In this chapter we discuss the different types of memory, their neurobiological basis, and disorders that affect these different systems and their clinical manifestations. In particular it is useful to distinguish between **long-term and working memory** (which is often erroneously referred to as short-term memory). While this distinction relates to the duration of a memory, it primarily refers to whether material is maintained in consciousness (***working memory***) or whether it may stored unconsciously and then retrieved into consciousness (***long-term memory***).

Working memory
Definition
This is defined as the limited capacity (around seven items or chunks of information) to store information in consciousness but that rapidly disappears when attention is diverted. A distinction is typically made between processes required for maintaining material and the control ('executive') processes required for manipulation of that material. Maintenance processes would typically be engaged by reciting a list of digits and requiring a subject to repeat them immediately (***digit span***). Executive control processes might be tested by requiring the subject to repeat the digits in reverse order.

Neurobiological basis and disorders of working memory
Studies in humans and monkeys have unequivocally demonstrated the importance of the lateral prefrontal cortex in working memory processes (see also Chapter 32). It has been suggested that different parts of the prefrontal cortex are important for the maintenance and control processes that constitute working memory. Other brain regions are clearly implicated in working memory processes in a modality-dependent way. Working memory for visuospatial material may rely upon occipitotemporal regions (when remembering, for example, the visual

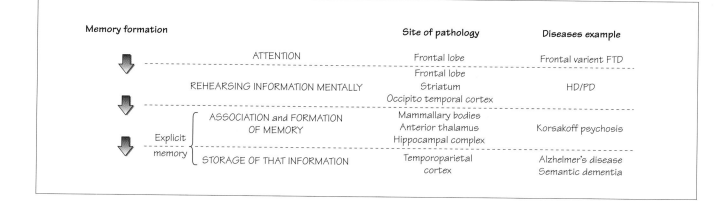

Memory formation		Site of pathology	Diseases example
ATTENTION		Frontal lobe	Frontal varient FTD
REHEARSING INFORMATION MENTALLY		Frontal lobe Striatum Occipito temporal cortex	HD/PD
Explicit memory	ASSOCIATION and FORMATION OF MEMORY	Mammallary bodies Anterior thalamus Hippocampal complex	Korsakoff psychosis
	STORAGE OF THAT INFORMATION	Temporoparietal cortex	Alzhelmer's disease Semantic dementia

properties of an object) or occipitoparietal regions (when remembering spatial properties). On the other hand, holding verbal or phonological material in working memory seems to require lateral temporal cortex. Whatever the domain, it appears that the efficient flexible use of working memory processes depends upon coordinated interactivity of frontal control processes and modality-dependent 'slave' systems.

Abnormalities in this system typically occur with damage in the sites listed above, especially the prefrontal cortex, as well as in some disorders of the basal ganglia (e.g. **Huntington's** and **Parkinson's disease**) where there is disruption of corticostriatal circuits (see Chapter 41). In these patients there is a difficulty in taking in information and as such the individuals have difficulty solving problems that require the ongoing manipulation of data.

Long-term memory
Definition
This is a store of practically unlimited capacity and the memories stored within this system may persist over a lifetime. Long-term memory is primarily divided in to **explicit** and **implicit** components.

Explicit memory refers to memories that are accessible to consciousness. It is divided into **episodic memory** (memory for episodes or events; typically, memory with an autobiographical content) and **semantic memory** (knowledge of facts; memory that is not characterized by an autobiographical content). Thus, an episodic memory of Paris might comprise the memory of a visit there, while a semantic memory is that Paris is the capital of France, situated on the Seine, etc.

Implicit memory refers to memory that is not accessible to consciousness and typically refers to motor memory; it encompasses the acquisition of **motor skills, conditioning** (e.g. Pavlov's dogs salivating when hearing a bell), as well as **priming**. This latter process is defined as the subject's ability to provide answers to general questions (e.g. the word 'Paris' when asked to name a city), even when they do not remember this prior exposure.

Neuroanatomical basis and disorders of long-term memory
The famous case of H.M., who suffered the removal of medial temporal cortices bilaterally (for intractable epilepsy), provided the first clear evidence that the episodic memory system depends upon medial regions of the temporal lobe. In addition, his case also highlighted the difference between explicit and implicit memories and the fact that different systems underlie episodic and semantic memory at the neuroanatomical level. Subsequent to his operation, H.M. was unable to learn or recall new episodes or experiences in his life. However, his ability to learn new motor skills was preserved as was his factual knowledge. While there is a great deal of evidence underpinning the importance of medial temporal structures, especially the hippocampus, in episodic memory processes, it is clear that, as with working memory processes, distributed brain systems, frequently requiring prefrontally mediated control, are necessary for optimum autobiographical memory processes (see Chapters 16 and 32). In this respect, patients with certain forms of neurodegenerative disorders with relatively widespread pathology may have profound disorders of long-term memory, as for example in **Alzheimer's disease** (see Chapter 57). In this condition there is pathology within the hippocampal and related structures (see Chapter 46) as well as temporal and parietal cortices and patients develop problems of anterograde memory (i.e. the laying down of new memories) followed by progressive problems with retrograde memory (the retrieval of preformed established memories). This distinction in anterograde and retrograde memories is thought to have a basis in the transferring of information from hippocampal structures to the overlying cortex and thus as the pathology spreads out so the memory processes are affected in a similar fashion. While in Alzheimer's disease the initial memory problem is more of an episodic nature, in some people there are problems within the semantic memory system. These cases of semantic dementia, wherein individuals begin to lose their knowledge of the meanings of words, depends upon damage to the inferior and lateral temporal cortex and is seen in some patients with a *frontotemporal dementia (FTD)*.

Emotion, motivation and drug addiction

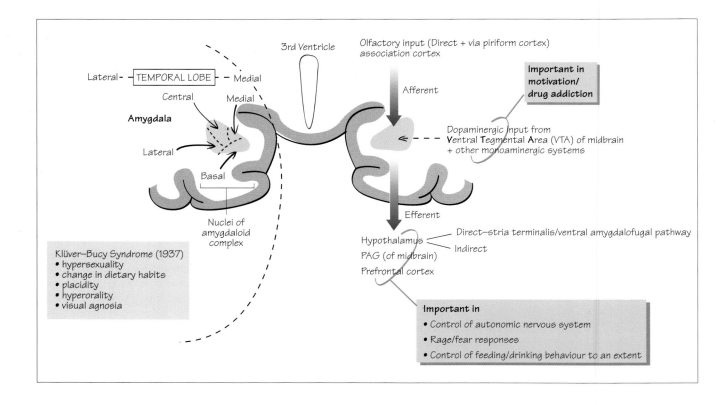

Lateral - TEMPORAL LOBE - Medial

Central — Medial

Amygdala

Lateral

Basal

Nuclei of amygdaloid complex

3rd Ventricle

Olfactory input (Direct + via piriform cortex) association cortex

Afferent

Important in motivation/ drug addiction

Dopaminergic input from Ventral Tegmental Area (VTA) of midbrain + other monoaminergic systems

Efferent

Hypothalamus — Direct—stria terminalis/ventral amygdalofugal pathway
PAG (of midbrain) — Indirect
Prefrontal cortex

Klüver–Bucy Syndrome (1937)
• hypersexuality
• change in dietary habits
• placidity
• hyperorality
• visual agnosia

Important in
• Control of autonomic nervous system
• Rage/fear responses
• Control of feeding/drinking behaviour to an extent

Emotion

The initial attempts to understand the brain bases of emotions focused upon the limbic system (see Chapter 46), with the **amygdala** as the key component in the system thought to be central to emotional processing. The evidence to support such an association has already been discussed in part (see Chapter 46), but it is also worth mentioning the *Klüver–Bucy syndrome*. This condition is seen with bilateral amygdala damage and is characterized by, among other phenomena, an apparent absence of the normal fear response and by marked placidity. In addition, functional neuroimaging studies in humans have been consistent with animal studies, implicating the amygdala in the processing of emotional stimuli and, notably, in fear conditioning (wherein a previously neutral stimulus can, through association with an unpleasant outcome, come to produce a fear response when presented alone). It is proposed that the amygdala is the critical site in which: (i) the necessary associations between the stimuli are formed using a process akin to the long-term potentiation (LTP) seen in the hippocampus (see Chapter 46); and (ii) the origin of the broad series of phenomena that constitute a fear response through its efferent projections.

Motivation

Emotions are potentially useful in that they are allied with, and perhaps consist of, behavioural responses: they may be critical in helping us to choose between competing behavioural possibilities and to guide behaviours that maximize rewarding and minimize punishing outcomes. The relationship between emotion and motivation is therefore an important one. In this respect, the dopamine systems, most notably the **mesolimbic system** (see also Chapter 55), which has connections with the amygdala, appear critical. A series of hypotheses have been put forward concerning the dopaminergic contribution to motivation.
• *Hedonia hypothesis*, in which dopamine is critical to the experience of pleasure. There is increasing evidence against this view.
• *Learning hypothesis*, in which dopamine is critical to learning the relationship between stimuli and rewards. In this theory dopamine acts as a 'teaching signal' for stimuli that predict rewards and thus is the origin of behaviour that makes the reward manifest.
• *Activation hypothesis*, in which dopamine is required for the actual engagement in work that must be done to obtain the reward. It is important for both the attentional and the locomotor components of the work involved in reward-seeking and consumption.
• *Incentive salience*, in which dopamine is important in imbuing certain stimuli with motivational or incentive properties.
It would be simplistic to express motivational processes solely in terms of the input of the mesolimbic dopamine system to the amygdala but it is nevertheless a useful model by which to explain drug addiction.

In addition to the motivational properties of specific stimuli, in many circumstances we must consider motivational states that appear stimulus independent. Feeding behaviours, for example, arise not solely from the motivational properties of foods (sight, smell, taste) but also from a drive state (hunger) dependent upon a number of homeostatic factors, for example endocrine signals (levels of insulin, and of the hormones leptin and ghrelin which, respectively, reduce and promote feeding behaviour) acting predominantly through the hypothalamus. A comprehensive description of a motivational state would require several levels of description together with an understanding of the interactions inherent in the state; for example, the extent to which motivational properties of stimuli themselves influence, and are influenced by, the drive state of the individual. A further important concern is when individuals are motivated towards behaviours that are at odds with their homoeostatic requirements and consequently detrimental to health, as is the case with addictive behaviours.

Drug addiction

Drugs are rewarding but the evidence is that addictive behaviours (and associated withdrawal phenomena) are determined by how the brain adapts in response to repeated drug administration rather than as a direct result of the fact that drugs may be intensely pleasurable. Conversely, although the reward properties of the drug are insufficient to explain addictive behaviours, it is simplistic, too, to consider addiction solely as behaviours aimed towards avoiding withdrawal symptoms. Rather, in addiction to considering addiction in terms of the pursuit of pleasurable states (drug-induced euphoria) or the avoidance of withdrawal states (an array of physical and psychological symptoms which may actually be produced simply by a stimulus or environment that has become associated with previous withdrawal), we must also take into account what may be considered a markedly augmented state of motivation to taking the drug—referred to as *craving*. Important in this respect is the fact that a craving may be precipitated by a drug-related stimulus or environment long after the individual has recovered from the withdrawal symptoms.

Other important phenomena that need to be explained are tolerance (a requirement for increased frequency and/or dose of the drug with repeated usage) and sensitization (in contrast to tolerance effects, some of the consequences of the drug may actually increase with repeated ingestion). Interestingly, neither tolerance nor sensitization are explicable in purely pharmacological terms because both phenomena also show certain features suggesting that they are conditioned responses. One view that has been put forward to account for the simultaneous occurrence of tolerance and sensitization is that while the pleasurable effects of the drug diminish with repeated administration (leading to tolerance), the drug and related environments and paraphernalia become, over time, more likely to capture attention and to precipitate the associated behaviours (sensitization).

While the neurobiological basis of drug addiction is still not fully understood, there is increasing evidence that it involves mesolimbic dopamine systems and genetic susceptibilities in genes which may in turn affect the normal functioning of this pharmacological system. A recent example of this is seen in some patients with *Parkinson's disease* who develop abnormal behaviours with their dopaminergic therapies which leads to them taking excessive amounts with consequent behavioural changes and actions—the so-called **dopamine dysregulation syndrome** which can involve pathological gambling and hypersexuality.

49 Neural plasticity and neurotrophic factors I: The peripheral nervous system

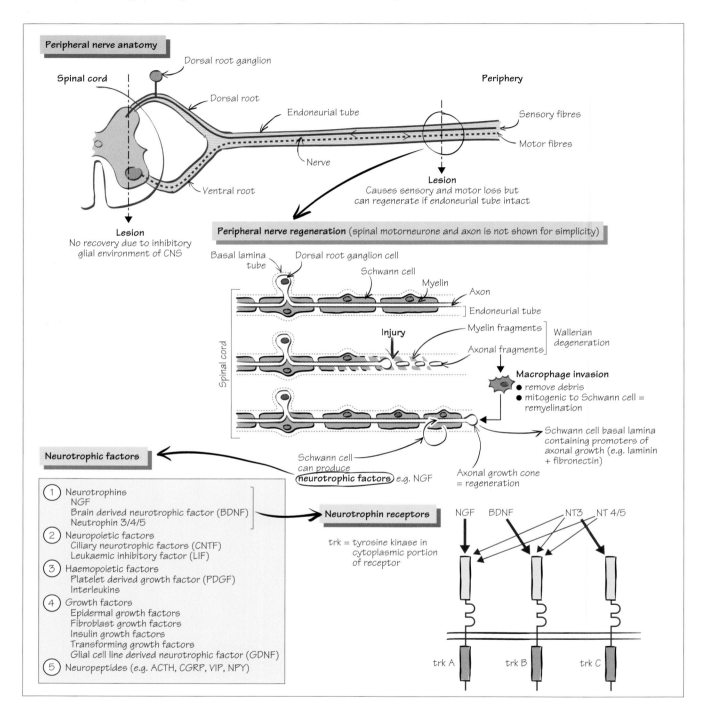

The peripheral nervous system (PNS) is capable of significant repair, to some extent independent of the age at which damage occurs. In contrast, the central nervous system (CNS) has always been thought of as being unable to repair itself although there is now mounting evidence that there is considerable plasticity within it even in the adult state and that most if not all areas of the CNS are capable of some degree of reorganization (see Chapter 50).

Repair in the peripheral nervous system

Injury to a peripheral nerve if severe enough will cause permanent damage with loss of sensation, loss of muscle bulk and weakness. However, in many cases the nerve is able to repair itself, as the peripheral axon can regrow under the influence of the favourable environment of the Schwann cells. This is in contrast to the CNS where the neuroglial cells (astrocytes and oligodendrocytes) are generally inhibitory to axonal growth, even though most CNS neurones are capable of growing new axons.

When a peripheral nerve is damaged, the distal aspect of the axon is lost by a process of **Wallerian degeneration**. Wallerian degeneration leads to the removal and recycling of both axonal and myelin-derived material, but leaves in place dividing Schwann cells inside the basal lamina tube that surrounds all nerve fibres. These columns of Schwann cells surrounded by basal lamina are known as **endoneurial tubes**, and provide the favourable substrate for axonal growth.

Following injury, the degenerating nerve fibre elicits an initial macrophage invasion and this in turn provides the mitogenic input to the Schwann cell. The regenerating axon starts to sprout within hours of injury and contacts the Schwann cell basal laminae on one side, and the Schwann cell membrane on the other. The Schwann cell basal lamina is especially important in the process of axonal sprouting as it contains a number of molecules that are powerful promoters of axonal outgrowth *in vitro* (e.g. laminin and fibronectin).

In addition to providing a favourable substrate for axonal growth, Schwann cells also produce a number of neurotrophic factors, including nerve growth factor (NGF; see below). Thus, the Schwann cell provides a substrate along which the regenerating axon can grow, as well as providing a favourable humoral neurotrophic environment. It also helps direct the regenerating axon back to its appropriate target, by means of the endoneurial tube. Occasionally, the regrowth of the axons is inaccurate or incomplete so, for example, following damage to the third cranial nerve one can have aberrant regeneration such that there is elevation of the eyelid on looking down.

In contrast to axonal damage, the loss of the cell body (in the ventral horn or dorsal root ganglia) leads to an irreversible and permanent loss of axons in the peripheral nerve. Examples of such disorders include *poliomyelitis* and *motorneurone disease (MND)* with respect to the α-MN, and a number of inflammatory and *paraneoplastic syndromes* in the case of the dorsal root ganglia (see Chapters 57 and 59). In all these cases the loss of axons is secondary to the loss of the cell body and so no regeneration is possible. Attempts to rescue dying α-MN in *MND* via the peripheral delivery of neurotrophic factors has been tried without much success to date (see Chapter 57).

Neurotrophic factors

The number of identified neurotrophic factors has expanded greatly since the original description of the first of these, NGF. These factors, many of which are also found to influence non-neural populations of cells, form discrete families that act through specific types of receptors. Many of these receptors are composed of subunits, one or some of which form common binding domains for a family of neurotrophic factors. For example, the neurotrophin family of neurotrophic factors and the *trk* receptors use a range of cytoplasmic tyrosine kinases as part of their signalling mechanism.

Many populations of neurones respond to neurotrophic factors experimentally both *in vitro* and in the lesioned animal. However, despite these encouraging results, the administration of neurotrophic factors to patients in clinical trials of neurodegenerative disorders and neuropathies has met with only limited success. This argues against these disorders being the result of specific neurotrophic factor deficiencies (see Chapter 57). More recently, greater success has been achieved with the direct infusion of neurotrophic factor into the brain parenchyma rather than using the cerebrospinal fluid (CSF) or periphery, e.g. glial cell line derived neurotrophic factor (GDNF) in Parkinson's disease (see Chapters 41 and 57).

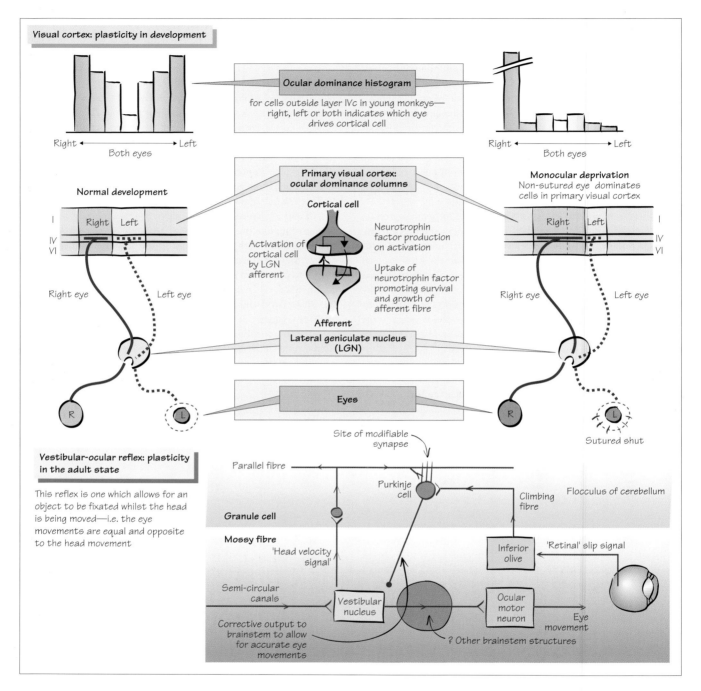

There is now mounting evidence that regeneration and reorganization can occur in the adult central nervous system (CNS). However, plasticity in the CNS is probably not due to a major production of new neurones, as most neurones in the mature CNS are postmitotic, but to their ability to extend branching new axons. The time at which this is most florid is in the early postnatal period when the systems of the brain are developing, and it is during this time that major modifications can be made.

The mechanisms underlying this plasticity are not fully known, but the production and uptake of factors promoting neuronal growth and survival (**neurotrophic factors**) are important.

Plasticity in the developing visual system

In their pioneering studies, Hubel and Wiesel demonstrated that at birth the input to laminae IV of the primary visual cortex (V1) is diffuse and that it is only during the **critical period** of development (in cats this is up to 3–14 weeks of postnatal life while in humans it may be several years) that these inputs segregate and form the basis of ocular dominance columns (see Chapter 27).

The segregation of input is dependent on the amount and type of activity within the afferent pathway from each eye; the greater this is, the more likely it is that the afferent input will gain control over those cortical neurones. Thus, ocular dominance (OD) columns will form in the absence of competition between the input from the two eyes but will not develop when there is no afferent input from either eye.

Hubel and Wiesel experimentally manipulated the inputs by initially depriving one eye of an input by suturing it shut (**monocular deprivation**) and then in later experiments by reversing the procedure (**'reverse suturing'**). Monocular deprivation created an expansion of the thalamic influence from the unsutured eye in layer IV with a subsequent shift in OD columns so that more cortical cells were under the control of the open eye. This pattern could be rapidly reversed by 'reverse suturing' during the critical period, which implies that the initial shift in thalamic influence on cortical cells is caused by the activation of synapses that were present but functionally suppressed as there is not enough time for any axonal outgrowth. However, in time the initially suppressed synapses from the uncompetitive eye would be physically lost as the active thalamic input takes over the control of cortical cells.

The correct segregation of the ocular inputs into V1 as OD columns is important for the generation of many of the other visual functions in V1. However, once outside the critical period the ability to modify the visual cortex in such a fashion is reduced, but not lost.

Plasticity in the adult state
Somatosensory system and the vestibulo-ocular reflex
It is now known that the somatosensory system is capable of being remodelled in the face of alterations in the input from the peripheral receptors. Thus, the loss of input from a digit (e.g. by amputation) does not lead to a permanently silent area of cortex, but instead the adjacent cortical areas with sensory inputs from adjacent digits would sprout axons and exert influence over this initially silent cortical area.

Conversely, increased afferent information in a sensory pathway results in an expansion of the cortical area receiving that input. Simplistically, it can be imagined that the activity in a given afferent induces the production of a neurotrophic factor in the postsynaptic cell, which then binds to the appropriate receptor in the active presynaptic terminal promoting its growth and survival. In this way the CNS is constantly remodelling itself based on the amount and type of ongoing afferent information.

Subsequently, it was discovered that major sensory deficits, such as the deafferentation of a whole limb, produced similar results which implied that the reclaiming of cortical areas by adjacent inputs was not solely achieved by the local sprouting of axons in the cortex.

Occasionally, this plasticity may go awry in certain situations, such as in **dystonia**. In this condition, abnormal plasticity in the primary motor and sensory cortices is thought to cause abnormal activation of muscles, this a resultant abnormal posturing of a body (see also Chapter 41). A further example of the plasticity of the mature CNS is seen with the vestibulo-ocular reflex (see Chapters 30 and 39). The vestibular system provides a signal to the CNS on head velocity and this is relayed to the cerebellum via mossy fibres. However, the other input to the cerebellum—the climbing fibre—can provide information on the degree to which the image is slipping across the retina (the degree to which eye movements are compensating or not for head movement). This input from the climbing fibre is not only important in providing a signal on the degree to which the reflex is working but also provides a critical input to correct it. Thus, if one alters the relationship between ocular and head movements by having the patient wear prisms, for example, the reflex adapts with time to compensate for the new relationship and this adaptation is possible because the climbing fibre input can modify the parallel fibre (and so indirectly mossy fibre) input to the Purkinje cell (see Chapter 39). The basis for this latter modification at the level of the Purkinje cell is an intracellular process and is termed **long-term depression** (**LTD**; see Chapter 39).

Neural stem cells
In many adult tissues, cell loss occurring through natural attrition or injury is balanced by the proliferation and subsequent differentiation of stem cells. In the adult CNS this was thought not to be the case, but recent evidence has shown that neural precursor cells are to be found in the mature CNS of mammals including humans. These cells are mainly found in the hippocampus and around the ventricles (in the subventricular zone) and appear to be able to form functionally active neurones. However, their role in plasticity and repair is unknown, but in the dentate gyrus of the hippocampus these cells may have a role in memory and mediating the effects of various hormones (e.g. cortisol/corticosterone) and drugs (e.g. antidepressants) on CNS function.

Limits on the regenerative capacity of the adult central nervous system
It must be realized that this regenerative capacity of the CNS is limited as:

1 neurones are postmitotic in the mature CNS, and the stem cell population is small and localized to certain sites; and
2 glial cells in the CNS are generally inhibitory to axonal outgrowth (see Chapter 4).

Astrocytes produce signals that stop axons growing and oligodendrocytes produce a number of factors that repel axons or even cause the approaching axonal growth cone to collapse. This often becomes more apparent at the time of the CNS insult, when glial cells divide, become activated and form a glial scar.

Examination of the nervous system

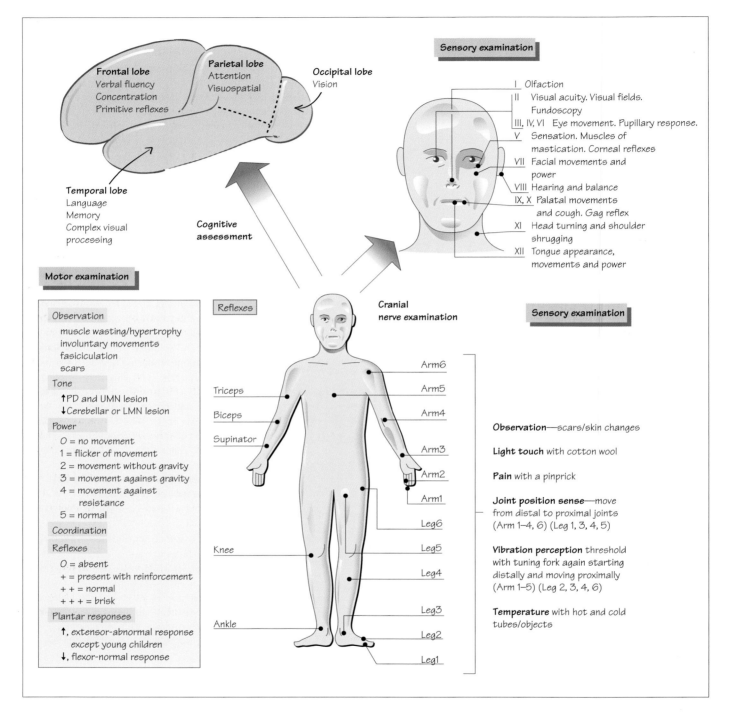

Frontal lobe
Verbal fluency
Concentration
Primitive reflexes

Parietal lobe
Attention
Visuospatial

Occipital lobe
Vision

Temporal lobe
Language
Memory
Complex visual
processing

Cognitive assessment

Sensory examination

I   Olfaction
II   Visual acuity. Visual fields. Fundoscopy
III, IV, VI   Eye movement. Pupillary response.
V   Sensation. Muscles of mastication. Corneal reflexes
VII   Facial movements and power
VIII   Hearing and balance
IX, X   Palatal movements and cough. Gag reflex
XI   Head turning and shoulder shrugging
XII   Tongue appearance, movements and power

Motor examination

Reflexes

Cranial nerve examination

Sensory examination

Observation
  muscle wasting/hypertrophy
  involuntary movements
  fasiciculation
  scars

Tone
  ↑PD and UMN lesion
  ↓Cerebellar or LMN lesion

Power
  0 = no movement
  1 = flicker of movement
  2 = movement without gravity
  3 = movement against gravity
  4 = movement against resistance
  5 = normal

Coordination

Reflexes
  0 = absent
  + = present with reinforcement
  + + = normal
  + + + = brisk

Plantar responses
  ↑, extensor-abnormal response except young children
  ↓, flexor-normal response

Triceps
Biceps
Supinator
Knee
Ankle

Arm6
Arm5
Arm4
Arm3
Arm2
Arm1
Leg6
Leg5
Leg4
Leg3
Leg2
Leg1

Observation—scars/skin changes

Light touch with cotton wool

Pain with a pinprick

Joint position sense—move from distal to proximal joints (Arm 1–4, 6) (Leg 1, 3, 4, 5)

Vibration perception threshold with tuning fork again starting distally and moving proximally (Arm 1–5) (Leg 2, 3, 4, 6)

Temperature with hot and cold tubes/objects

The examination of the nervous system can be broken down into a number of separate assessments.

Cognitive examination

General

Orientation in time, person and place: if this can not be correctly answered (assuming the patient has no major language deficits) then the patient is either acutely confused or severely demented, in which case the remainder of the cognitive examination is unlikely to be helpful.

Frontal lobe function

Verbal fluency: number of words generated beginning with a certain letter (e.g. 's') or specific category (e.g. animals) over a 60- or 90-s period. The latter task also relies on an intact temporoparietal cortex.

Concentration: the ability to take in and repeat back immediately a list of objects or a name and address.

Primitive reflexes: including pouting of the lips when they are tapped and grasping the examiner's hand when it is gently moved across the patient's hand.

Parietal lobe function

Attention: or neglect of visual or somatosensory stimuli in the contra-lateral sensory hemifield.

Dyspraxia: the patient is unable to form, copy or mime gestures and common tasks (e.g. combing hair).

Visuospatial function: the ability to copy drawings (e.g. interlocking pentagons).

Temporal lobe function

Anterograde memory: the ability to remember a standard name and address given to the patient (e.g. Peter Marshall, 42 Market Street, Chelmsford, Essex) 5 min after it has been given and retained. It is though important to ensure that the name and address has been remembered in the first place because sometimes patients with frontal lobe damage do badly on this test as they cannot take in the initial name and address because of poor attention.

Language: language assessment involves listening to spontaneous speech for content and fluency, naming objects, repeating phrases (e.g. 'no ifs, ands or buts'), following commands, reading and writing.

Cranial nerves

Olfactory nerve: each nostril is tested separately with a range of standard odours, avoiding ammonia as a testing solution as it irriates the nose and thus activates the trigeminal (not olfactory) system.

Optic nerve: visual acuity for each eye is tested using standard eyesight charts. The visual fields for each eye are then tested with examination of the blind spot if necessary (see Chapter 26). The fundi (back of the eye) are examined with an ophthalmoscope looking for abnormalities of the retina and optic disc, e.g. swollen (papilloedema) or pale and atrophic (optic atrophy). Colour vision (using the Ishihara colour plates) and pupillary responses can also be tested.

Oculomotor, trochlear and abducens nerve: ptosis and pupillary abnormalities are looked for (e.g. Horner's syndrome; see Chapter 16). The eye movements in all directions are then tested and the patient reports any diplopia (see Chapter 42).

Trigeminal nerve: sensation is tested in all three divisions of the trigeminal nerve and the power of the jaw muscles. In some cases the corneal reflex is tested by lightly touching the cornea with cotton wool. The patient should respond quickly by rapidly blinking; if not, it is worth checking the patient is not wearing contact lenses as this can give a false positive for the loss of the corneal reflex.

Facial nerve: the power of facial muscles is tested, e.g. the patient screws up their eyes tightly, blows out their cheeks or purses their lips. The examiner should *not* be able to overcome any of these movements.

Vestibulocochlear nerve: hearing is tested in each ear by gently whispering a number into each. More formal testing can be performed with tuning forks.

Glossopharyngeal and vagus nerve: the patient opens their mouth wide and says 'ahhhhhh' to assess movement of the palate. The gag reflex can be tested where a spatula is gently placed against the posterior pharyngeal wall and reflex movement of the palate seen. Testing the strength and character of a cough can also be helpful in some cases.

Spinal accessory nerve: tested by getting the patient to turn their head to the right and left and shrug their shoulders. The examiner should not be able to overcome this movement.

Hypoglossal nerve: tested by looking at the tongue in the floor of the mouth for wasting or fasciculation; it is then protruded from the mouth and any deviation from the midline noted. Power is tested by getting the patient to push the tongue into each cheek, assuming they do not have any significant facial weakness.

Motor system examination of the limbs

The examination of the motor system should include the following.

Observation: involuntary movements, wasting, weakness, fasciculation, scars or deformities.

Tone: the limb is gently moved and the stiffness of it assessed. It is increased in Parkinson's disease or upper motorneurone (UMN) lesions and decreased in lower motorneurone (LMN) or cerebellar lesions (see Chapters 34–36). Sometimes the tone is increased because the patient cannot relax or is in pain.

Power: movements are assessed and scored according to the MRC rating scale (see figure).

Coordination: the ability to coordinate movements in the upper limb is tested by getting the patient to touch the examiner's finger and then their own nose as the finger is slowly moved around in space. This may be abnormal if there is weakness, sensory loss or cerebellar disease. Alternatively, in the upper limb the patient can be asked to rapidly pronate and supinate their hand. In the lower limb, coordination is tested by getting the patient to walk normally, then heel–toe walking and finally by getting the patient while lying down to run their right/left heel along their left/right shin, respectively.

Reflexes: these are tested by tapping the tendons at certain sites in the upper and lower limb. Reflexes can be absent, reduced, normal or brisk. The latter implies a UMN lesion while reduced or absent reflexes implies a dysfunction in part of the spinal monosynaptic reflex (see Chapter 35), assuming the patient's muscles are properly relaxed.

Plantar responses: the sole of the foot is gently scratched along its lateral aspect and the toes should fan out and the big toe go down (flexor or normal plantar response). If the toes point up and this is not a withdrawal response, then this implies a UMN lesion.

Sensory examination

Sensation in the limbs is tested at the extremities and in the dermatomes using a number of tests.

Light touch: cotton wool is gently applied to the skin, having checked that the patient can feel it normally (test on face first, assuming there is no trigeminal sensory loss).

Pinprick: using a blunted pin (which is *not* reusable). Do not use needles as these are too sharp.

Temperature: using cold and hot tubes or objects.

Vibration perception threshold (VPT): using a tuning fork applied to the distal interphalangeal joint or big toe. The patient must feel it vibrating and *not* just feel it being applied to the joint. If this is not felt to vibrate, it is moved proximally.

Joint position sense (JPS): tested by slightly moving the terminal joint in the hand or toe, having checked that the patient understands what is meant by up and down movements. This movement should be very slight, as JPS is very sensitive in humans. If the movement cannot be detected then larger movements are made at these joints before moving to more proximal joints, in the same way as for VPT.

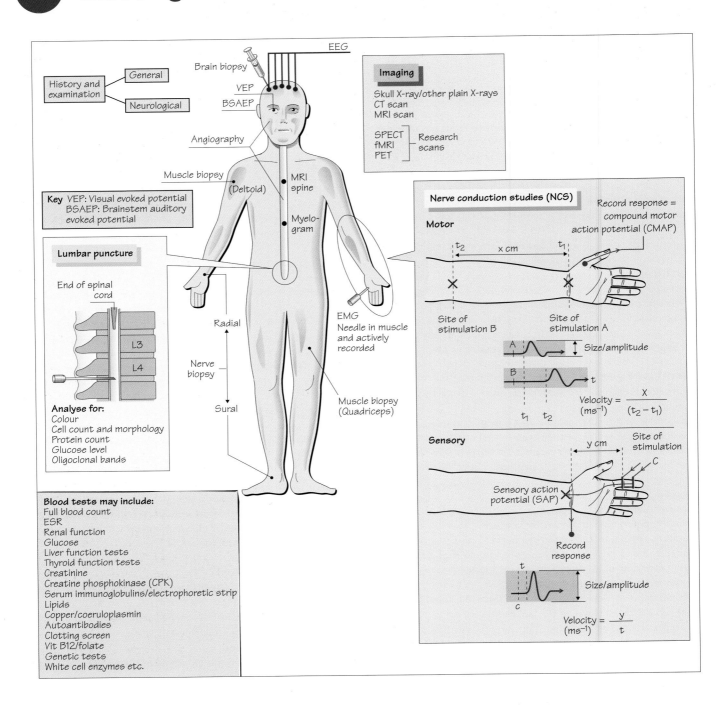

EEG

Brain biopsy

VEP

BSAEP

History and examination — General, Neurological

Angiography

Muscle biopsy (Deltoid)

Key VEP: Visual evoked potential
BSAEP: Brainstem auditory evoked potential

MRI spine

Myelo-gram

Imaging

Skull X-ray/other plain X-rays
CT scan
MRI scan

SPECT
fMRI — Research scans
PET

Lumbar puncture

End of spinal cord

L3
L4

Analyse for:
Colour
Cell count and morphology
Protein count
Glucose level
Oligoclonal bands

Radial

Nerve biopsy

Sural

EMG
Needle in muscle and actively recorded

Muscle biopsy (Quadriceps)

Blood tests may include:
Full blood count
ESR
Renal function
Glucose
Liver function tests
Thyroid function tests
Creatinine
Creatine phosphokinase (CPK)
Serum immunoglobulins/electrophoretic strip
Lipids
Copper/coeruloplasmin
Autoantibodies
Clotting screen
Vit B12/folate
Genetic tests
White cell enzymes etc.

Nerve conduction studies (NCS)

Record response = compound motor action potential (CMAP)

Motor

t_2 x cm t_1

Site of stimulation B   Site of stimulation A

A — Size/amplitude
B — t

t_1 t_2 t_1 t_2

$$\text{Velocity} = \frac{X}{(t_2 - t_1)} \ (\text{ms}^{-1})$$

Sensory

y cm   Site of stimulation

C

Sensory action potential (SAP)

Record response

t — Size/amplitude
c

$$\text{Velocity} = \frac{y}{t} \ (\text{ms}^{-1})$$

The investigation of the nervous system involves a number of specialist procedures as well as a series of standard tests. However, the key to investigating any patient is through their history and examination, as this will highlight the likely nature and site of the problem. In this chapter the major investigative procedures available in patients with neurological problems are presented, along with their indications.

History and examination

History and examination detail the problem, its evolution and other relevant medical history along with the results of the neurological examination (see Chapter 51).

Blood tests

A large number of tests are available (see figure for examples).

Imaging (see also Chapter 53)

• Plain X-rays are rarely of value in the diagnosis of neurological disease, unless one suspects the patient has a related disease in another site such as the chest (e.g. lung cancer).

- Computerized tomography (CT) gives detailed X-ray images of the brain, skull and lower spine. It is useful for diagnosing structural lesions such as tumours, major strokes or skull fractures. It is widely available but has limited resolution especially in the posterior fossa and cervicothoracic spinal cord.
- Magnetic resonance imaging (MRI) is a noisy claustrophobic procedure which relies on patient cooperation. It provides detailed images of all parts of the brain and spinal cord and the use of different sequences has increased its utility and diagnostic strength. It does not involve any radiation.
- Magnetic resonance angiography and venography (MRA/MRV) scans delineate the major blood vessels to, within and from the brain. They are primarily used to look for significant narrowing (stenosis) of the extracranial carotid arteries in the neck, aneurysms in the brain and blockage of the major venous sinuses in the brain, but are not as sensitive as angiography.
- Angiography involves the passing of a small catheter to the origin of the major blood vessels of the brain (both carotid and vertebral arteries), and a small amount of dye is injected. The dye can then be followed using a video and images captured rapidly over time as the dye passes through the vascular tree. The procedure is invasive and carries a small risk of complication, but is useful in accurately delineating any vascular abnormality (e.g. carotid stenoses, aneurysms, arteriovenous malformations and venous sinus thrombosis). It can also be used to look for specific vascular abnormalities in the spinal cord.
- Myelography is rarely used nowadays to delineate abnormalities in the spinal cord because of the non-invasiveness and resolution of MRI. However, it can be helpful in some circumstances and involves injecting a radio-opaque dye via a lumbar puncture into the subarachnoid space around the spine.
- Single photon emission computed tomography (SPECT) involves radioactive isotopes which typically provide information on perfusion within the brain. It has low resolution.
- Functional MRI (fMRI) is a research tool that measures activation of brain regions during tasks performed in the scanner by assessing oxygen uptake.
- Positron emission tomography (PET) detects the release of positrons from specific substances that bind to certain chemical sites within the brain. It is only used for research purposes.

Electrical tests

- Electrocardiography (ECG) is an electrical recording from the heart, and is performed in many patients with neurological disease, especially those with muscle disease, blackouts or some genetic disorders.
- Electroencephalography (EEG) measures the electrical activity and rhythms of the brain and is helpful in patients with decreased levels of consciousness, epilepsy (see Chapter 58) and some patients with sleep disorders (e.g. narcolepsy; see Chapter 44).
- Nerve conduction studies (NCS) involve stimulating both sensory and motor nerves and measuring the response. The general principle is that one stimulates at one site of the nerve and records at another or the muscle it innervates. The size and speed of the response are important. Loss of myelin (demyelination) slows the speed of conduction, while a loss of axons gives a smaller response but normal conduction velocity. It is useful in determining whether the patient has a neuropathy, what type (demyelinating vs. axonal) and the extent (focal or generalized).
- Electromyography (EMG) involves placing a needle into the muscle

and recording the electrical activity within it. It is useful in the diagnosis of muscle disease and in patients with motorneuronal loss as occurs in motorneurone disease (**MND**), because EMG can show the extent of denervation which may help in the diagnosis.
- Evoked potentials (EPs) can be in the visual pathway (visual-evoked potential or responses; VEP), auditory pathway (brainstem auditory-evoked potential) or peripheral nerves in the arms or legs (somatosensory-evoked potential). The test involves stimulating the peripheral receptor (eye, ear or median/posterior tibial nerve) and measuring the cortical response. This gives a measure of conduction along the pathway that has both a peripheral and CNS component. The most commonly used test is VEP in *multiple sclerosis* looking for asymptomatic demyelination in the visual pathways.
- Central motor conduction time (CMCT) measures the time from stimulating the motor cortex to measuring a muscle response in the periphery such as the hand. It is not routinely available and can be used as a measure of integrity of the descending corticospinal tract assuming that there is no dysfunction within the peripheral motor apparatus.
- Thermal thresholds is a subjective test designed to look at small fibre responses in patients. It relies on the patient detecting changes in temperature in the hands and feet. It is not routinely available in most centres.

Cerebrospinal fluid analysis

Cerebrospinal fluid (CSF) can be obtained from a number of sites but is routinely obtained by a lumbar puncture, which involves passing a small needle into the subarachnoid space in the lower lumbar spine. CSF should be clear and the opening pressure is measured before three separate tubes of fluid are sent for analysis to include the following.
- Number and type of cells, typically raised in infections (e.g. **meningitis** and **encephalitis**) as well as in **malignant meninigitis** (where cancer cells seed themselves along the meninges).
- Culture of the CSF to look for infective organisms, including a Gram stain in meningitis and PCR for the causative organism in some infections of the CNS (e.g. herpes simplex virus in herpes encephalitis).
- Glucose, which can be low in certain types of infection or meningitis and metastatic tumours growing in the meninges.
- Protein, which can be raised in some types of neuropathy, tumour and in lesions causing a block to spinal CSF flow.
- Oligoclonal bands indicative of immunoglobulin synthesis specifically within the CNS, typically seen in **multiple sclerosis**.

Nerve/muscle biopsy

In cases where there is evidence of nerve or muscle disease, a biopsy may be helpful in identifying the defect more specifically. Typical sites are the radial and sural nerves and the quadriceps and deltoid muscles.

Brain biopsy

This is routinely performed in patients with brain tumours to confirm the diagnosis and to some extent predict prognosis. In some cases of progressive neurological disease for which no obvious cause can be found, a biopsy looking specifically for inflammation in the blood vessels (vasculitis) as well as prion disease may be considered. However, in the latter case, strict guidelines must be followed with respect to the reuse/disposal of the instruments.

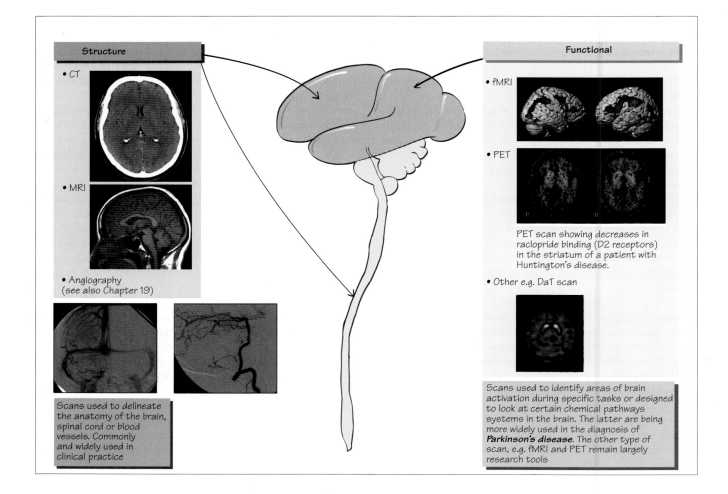

Structure
- CT
- MRI
- Angiography (see also Chapter 19)

Scans used to delineate the anatomy of the brain, spinal cord or blood vessels. Commonly and widely used in clinical practice

Functional
- fMRI
- PET

PET scan showing decreases in raclopride binding (D2 receptors) in the striatum of a patient with Huntington's disease.

- Other e.g. DaT scan

Scans used to identify areas of brain activation during specific tasks or designed to look at certain chemical pathways systems in the brain. The latter are being more widely used in the diagnosis of **Parkinson's disease**. The other type of scan, e.g. fMRI and PET remain largely research tools

Imaging of the central nervous system (CNS) is essentially designed to look either at structure (computed tomography [CT], magnetic resonance imaging [MRI], angiography) or function (functional MRI [fMRI], positron emission tomography [PET], and single photon emission CT [SPECT]). In clinical practice it is the former that is the mainstay of practice, with the latter tests reserved for patients being investigated for specific problems or as part of a research project. In general structural scanning is undertaken to determine the following:
- Is there any abnormality in the CNS on imaging?
- If there is an abnormality, where is it and does it fit with the history and clinical examination?
- What is the likely nature of that abnormality pathologically based on its radiological appearance?

This information can be used for the future investigation and management of patients with neurological disorders. In this chapter we will outline the major imaging modalities used in clinical practice, their indications, value and drawbacks.

Structural imaging
Computed tomography imaging
Basic principle: this technique uses X-rays to scan the brain or lumbar spine and then reconstruct an image of that structure; it can be per-

formed with or without a contrast agent, the latter being used to better define blood vessels and abnormalities in the blood–brain barrier.

Use: imaging of the brain looking for major abnormalities, in particular stroke, head trauma, hydrocephalus or tumour, especially in the acute medical situation. It can also be used to look for skull fractures and prolapsed intervertebral discs in the lumbar spine, and in some cases can be used to look for cerebral aneurysms.

Advantages: widely available, and often gives useful and vital information especially in acute situations. It is very well tolerated by nearly all patients, even those who cannot fully cooperate, and if a general anaesthetic is needed to image the patient this is more easily performed with CT than MRI

Disadvantage: has poor contrast resolution compared to MRI and as such is not so good at identifying lesions in the posterior fossa and cervicothoracic spine, especially as there is often a lot of artefact with CT imaging and the posterior fossa from dental fillings.

Magnetic resonance imaging
Basic principle: this technique places the patient in a strong magnetic field which is then subject to a series of magnetic perturbations (scan sequence) which alters the orientation of hydrogen ions, such that their

change and subsequent shift back to normal position is detected. Thus, it does not use X-rays and is very sensitive to subtle changes in water content, which makes it a highly sensitive scan.

Use: most patients with neurological problems should have an MRI scan given its superior spatial resolution compared with CT scanning and the fact that any part of the neuroaxis can be scanned using it. Thus, it is used in patients with chronic neurological problems (e.g. multiple sclerosis) as well as those with evolving acute disorders (e.g. herpes encephalitis). It can also be used with a contrast agent (gadolinium) and to image blood vessels both on the arterial side (magnetic resonance angiography [MRA]) looking for carotid artery disease or intracerebral aneurysms and on the venous side (magnetic resonance venography [MRV]) looking especially for major venous sinus thromboses.

Advantages: high spatial resolution and the fact that any part of the neural axis can be imaged, along with the major vessels, without recourse to X-ray exposure or invasive procedures.

Disadvantage: it is a noisy, claustrophobic experience and requires the patient to be cooperative to some extent. Some patients cannot cope with the claustrophobia while agitated patients will move in the scanner causing major artefacts on the images. It also cannot be used in patients who contain metallic magnetic material such as a cardiac pacemaker.

Angiography

Basic principle: this is the imaging of blood vessels and it can be carried out using CT and MRI, but in some cases it requires the direct visualization of blood vessels using a radiolucent contrast agent injected into an artery with video fluroscopy to follow its course. Thus, the flow of the dye can be followed through the vasculature and X-rays taken to capture various different phases of the injection; this can identify problems on the arterial and venous sides of the circulation.

Use: its main value is the identification of vascular abnormalities such as aneurysms, arteriovenous malformations and venous sinus disease. In all cases angiography is either performed to confirm an equivocal MRA/MRV result or as a prelude to a more invasive procedure to deal with the underlying abnormality such as the obliteration of vascular malformations through intravascular occlusion techniques (gluing or coiling).

Advantage: it is the most high-resolution scan for identifying vascular abnormalities and is essential if intravascular interventional therapies are being considered.

Disadvantage: it is an invasive procedure with a small but nevertheless real complication rate of stroke and local haemorrhage/haematoma at the site at which the catheter is passed into the artery (typically the femoral artery in the groin).

Functional scanning

This embraces SPECT, PET and fMRI. Although there are a number of different types of scan, they can be thought of as looking at either:

• Blood flow/metabolism using glucose and oxygen markers to reflect neuronal activity and pathology, such that a loss of activity reflects an area that contains dysfunctional or dead neurons. So, for example, in Alzheimer's disease there will be hypoperfusion in the parietotemporal cortices. Such 'metabolic' scans can be undertaken for diagnostic and therapeutic purposes in some patients in routine clinical practice. Another related approach, which is currently only used in research, relies on looking at oxygen extraction in areas of the brain while the patient is being tested on a particular task with them actually lying in the MRI scanner being imaged. The resultant scan will show which areas of the brain are activated by that task. This is called fMRI, and has been used, for example, to see which areas of cortex are activated by specific types of cognitive or visual processing tasks.

• Specific neurochemical markers which are used to identify and label particular aspects of a neurotransmitter pathway. In Parkinson's disease this may involve looking at the dopamine transporter (e.g. DAT scans) or certain types of dopamine receptor (e.g. 11C-raclopride labelling of D2 receptors in PET). The former types of scan are found in many nuclear medicine departments and are widely available, while PET scanning is still only an experimental tool and found in a few research centres.

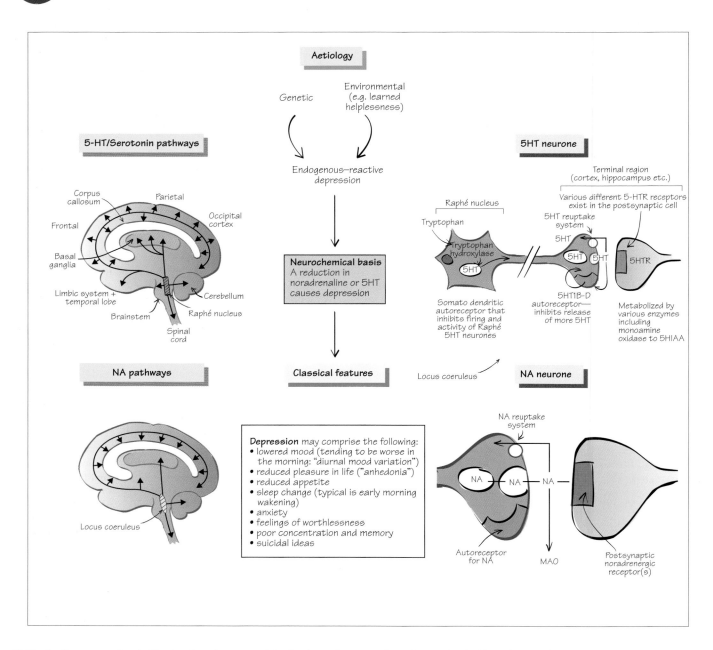

'Affect' refers to mood and affective disorders comprising both a pathological lowering (*depression*) and elevation (*mania*) of mood. Bipolar affective disorder (manic-depression) refers to an oscillation between depression and mania. These conditions are not simply characterized by mood changes, however, and depression may comprise a number of characteristic features.

Clinical features of affective disorders

Depression may comprise the following:
• lowered mood (tending to be worse in the morning: 'diurnal mood variation');
• reduced pleasure in life ('anhedonia');
• reduced appetite;
• sleep change (typically early morning wakening);
• anxiety;
• feelings of worthlessness;
• poor concentration and memory; and
• suicidal ideas.

   Mania is characterized by:
• elevated mood;
• grandiose ideas and actions;
• increased energy and feelings of well-being; and
• overactivity with reduced sleep.

   Both conditions may be accompanied by features of psychosis (delusions and hallucinations; see Chapter 55). The nature of the psychosis tends to be mood-congruent: in depression, the patient may believe that he or she is guilty of something or hear voices that are critical and unpleasant. Mania may be accompanied by grandiose delusions.

Depression
Aetiology
This is a common disorder with a lifetime prevalence that has been estimated to be as high as 15%, with women affected more than men (approximately 2 : 1). It can occur in response to adverse circumstances (**reactive depression**), as well as for no apparent circumstantial reason (**endogenous depression**), although often the distinction between these two different types of depression is not that clear-cut. In both cases the depression probably arises through a combination of genetic and environmental factors:

• Genetic: while a number of genes have been implicated in affective disorders, specific genes for depression have not been identified, so it is thought to have a polygenic component—which is maybe more significant in patients with bipolar disorders.

• Environmental and psychological factors are also extremely important. Background personality factors have been implicated as have social stressors, which have been hypothesized to produce depression by inducing in individuals a sense that they have no personal control over events in their lives (akin to **learned helplessness** in rats). This basic psychological model has been extended and superseded by the view that 'depressive cognitions' are fundamental to depression. That is, because an individual holds specific beliefs and attibutional styles, then he or she may be more vulnerable to the development of a depressive illness. This view is central to the emerging use of cognitive therapies in depression.

Neurochemical basis of depression
The **monoamine theory of depression** suggests that the illness is caused by reduced monoamine transmission. It derives from the observation that the tricyclic antidepressants—remarkably effective in the treatment of the illness—upregulate monaminergic transmission. However, the direct evidence for monoamine disturbance in depression is scant and inconsistent.

The **serotonin hypothesis** suggests that depression is linked to reduced serotoninergic function and gains support from the antidepressant efficacy of the newer generation of treatments: the selective serotonin reuptake inhibitors (SSRIs). Furthermore, temporary depletion of tryptophan (a precursor of serotonin) levels causes a transient but profound resurgence of depressive symptoms in people who have been successfully treated with SSRIs and in people with a depressive illness in remission.

Cognition in depression
Depression is associated with impairments or changes in performance on a number of tests of cognitive function. Memory deficits are prominent and occur across memory domains (working memory and episodic memory; see Chapter 47) and across modalities (verbal and visuospatial). Psychomotor retardation is also common with depressed people showing an apparent lack of motivation (see Chapter 48) and marked slowing of speech and motor functions, the latter manifest in generally slowed reaction times. Sustained attention may be poor as may planning and problem-solving. Interestingly, some of the changes in memory and attention are characterized by an interaction with the emotional nature of test material. For example, patients may preferentially remember or attend to stimuli that have negative connotations. They may also be more likely to perceive neutral stimuli as being emotionally negative.

Treatment
A number of different therapies are employed for the treatment of depression, and while these include **psychotherapy** and **electroconvulsive therapy (ECT)**, the most commonly used approach is with **antidepressant drugs**. Most of the drugs used in the treatment of depression inhibit the reuptake of norepinephrine and/or serotonin (5-HT). Less commonly used drugs are monoamine oxidase inhibitors (MAOIs). Because both uptake inhibitors and MAOIs increase the amount of norepinephrine and/or 5-HT in the synaptic cleft and so enhance the action of these transmitters, it was argued that depression resulted from an 'underactivity' of these monoaminergic systems (see above). In mania and bipolar affective disorders lithium has a mood-stabilizing action. **Lithium** salts have a low therapeutic : toxic ratio and adverse effects are common. **Carbamazapine** and **valproate** also have mood-stabilizing actions and can be used in cases of non-response or intolerance to lithium. The mechanisms involved in the mood-stabilizing effects of these drugs are unknown.

Amine uptake inhibitors
Tricyclic antidepressants (e.g. **imipramine, amitriptyline**) have proven antidepressant actions but no one drug has greater efficacy. The choice of drug is determined by the most acceptable or desired side-effects. For example, some have sedative actions (e.g. **amitriptyline, dosulepin**) and are more useful for agitated and anxious patients (see Chapter 56). Withdrawn and apathetic patients may benefit from less sedative drugs (e.g. **imipramine, lofepramine**). In addition to blocking amine uptake, the tricyclics block muscarinic receptors, α-adrenoreceptors and H1-histamine receptors. These actions frequently cause dry mouth, blurred vision, constipation, urinary retention, tachycardia and postural hypotension. In overdosage, the anticholinergic activity and a quinidine-like action may cause cardiac arrhythmias and sudden death (cardiotoxicity).

Some newer drugs (SNRIs), e.g. **venlafaxine**, inhibit the reuptake of serotonin and noradrenaline but lack the antimuscarinic and sedative effects of the tricyclics.

Drugs that selectively inhibit serotonin re-uptake (SSRIs) (e.g. **fluoxetine**) are less sedative, do not have the troublesome autonomic side-effects of the tricyclics and are safer in overdoses. However, they have their own spectrum of adverse effects, the most common being nausea, vomiting, diarrhoea and constipation. They may also cause sexual dysfunction.

Monoamine oxidase inhibitors
The older MAOIs (e.g. phenelzine) are irreversible non-selective inhibitors of monoamine oxidase (MAO). Their efficacy is similar to that of the tricyclics. They are rarely used now because of their adverse effects (postural hypotension, dizziness, anticholinergic effects and liver damage). Also there may be potentially serious interactions with sympathomimetic amines (e.g. ephedrine), often present in cough mixtures and decongestive medicines, or food containing tyramine (e.g. game, cheese). Tyramine is normally metabolized by MAO in the liver. If the enzyme is inhibited, the tyramine enters the circulation and displaces noradrenaline from sympathetic nerve terminals. This may cause severe hypertension and even stroke.

Moclobemide is a newer drug that selectively inhibits MAO_A and lacks most of the unwanted effects of non-selective MAOIs.

Atypical antidepressants
These drugs have little, if any, effect on serotonin or noradrenaline reuptake and do not inhibit MAO. Mirtazapine and trazodone are sedative antidepressants but have few autonomic effects. Because they are less cardiotoxic than the tricyclics they are less dangerous in overdosage.

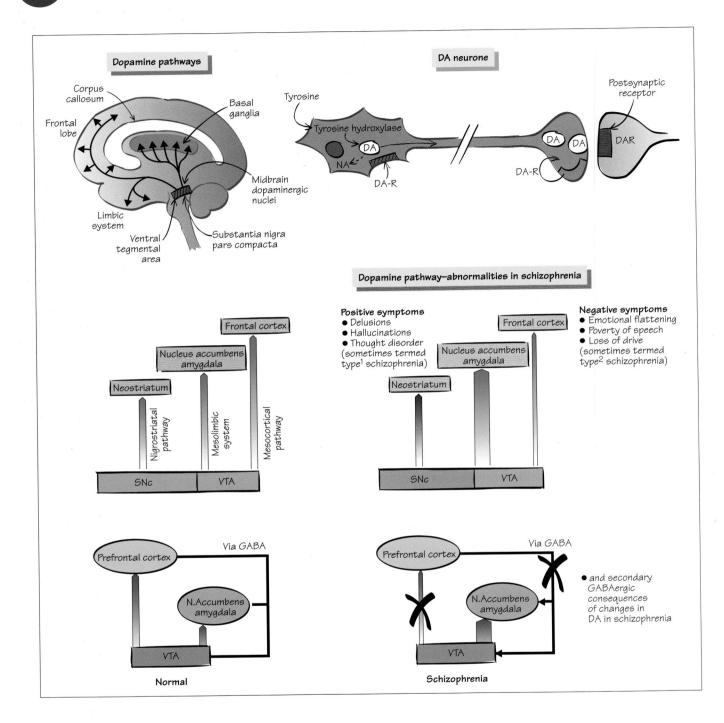

Schizophrenia is a syndrome characterized by specific psychological manifestations, including auditory hallucinations, delusions, thought disorders and behavioural disturbances. It is a common disorder with a lifetime prevalence of 1% and an incidence of 2–4 new cases per year per 10,000 population. It is more common in men and typically presents early in life. Like all psychiatric disorders there is no diagnostic test for this condition, which is defined by the existence of key symptoms.

Positive symptoms
• Delusions: abnormal or irrational beliefs, held with great conviction and out of keeping with an individual's sociocultural background.
• Hallucinations: perceptions in the absence of stimuli.
Negative symptoms
• Blunting of mood, apparent apathy, lack of spontaneous speech and action.
Disordered speech

Aetiology

A distinction used to be made between type 1 and 2 schizophrenia but this has fallen out of fashion as it may relate more to the length of time that the individual has had the condition. The cause of schizophrenia is unknown but a number of aetiological factors have been identified:

- Genetic: first-degree relatives of people with schizophrenia have a greatly increased risk of developing the disease; around 10% for siblings, 6% for parents and 13% for children. Concordance rates in twins are relatively high with figures that vary from 42% to 50% for monozygotic twins and between 0 and 14% for dizygotic twins.
- Environmental factors also have a substantial role with adoption studies demonstrating the importance of both genetic and environmental factors. In these studies gene–environment interactions have been demonstrated in children of schizophrenic parents adopted into good versus disturbed adoptive families. In this latter respect one influential theory relating to a family cause appeals to high levels of 'expressed emotion' (hostility, lack of emotional warmth, overinvolvement) as a risk for relapse.

The dopamine hypothesis of schizophrenia
Basic model

Simply stated, this embodies the idea that schizophrenia is caused by up-regulation of activity in the mesolimbic dopamine system. The evidence for this theory comes from the following observations:

- Dopamine-blocking drugs show an antipsychotic effect.
- Drugs that up-regulate dopamine can produce positive symptoms of psychosis (e.g. amphetamines).
- Some neuroimaging studies in patients have found evidence of dopamine up-regulation.

The dopamine hypothesis has been criticized for the lack of direct evidence in its favour and for certain inconsistencies: dopamine agonists do not produce all of the symptoms of schizophrenia (notably, they do not produce negative symptoms); dopamine-blocking drugs do not act immediately—there may be a long period before symptoms begin to resolve, which is not consistent with a simple view that these symptoms are caused by dopamine up-regulation.

Revised model

This has led to a revision of the original hypothesis, in particular both dopamine up-regulation and down-regulation must be invoked to account for the core features of the schizophrenia, with the positive symptoms arising from up-regulation of mesolimbic dopamine function and the negative symptoms from down-regulation of mesocortical function.

However, many still feel that is an inadequate explantation of this complex disorder and there is a view that schizophrenia is associated with **N-methyl-D-aspartate (NMDA) (glutamate) receptor hypofunction**. This arose from observations that NMDA blockers such as phencyclidine ('Angel Dust') and ketamine (widely used in anaesthesia) produce a psychotic state (including negative symptoms) that is held to be more strongly redolent of schizophrenia than the psychosis produced by dopaminergic agents. Therefore, it has been proposed that glutamate hypofunction may account for both up-regulation of the mesolimbic dopamine system, from a diminished excitatory drive of GABAergic inhibition (i.e. an attenuation of the 'brake' system), and down-regulation of the mesocortical system because of diminished direct drive (the 'activating' system).

Cognition in schizophrenia

It is important to note that, while schizophrenia is traditionally described in terms of psychotic symptoms, there is increasing evidence of cognitive deficits, particularly in the memory domain, that may accompany (and perhaps precede) the onset of these symptoms.

Treatment

The mainstay of therapy in schizophrenia remains the use of drugs that block dopamine receptors, of which there are at least five subtypes in the brain (D1–D5 receptors; see Appendix 1). These agents (e.g. chlorpromazine) are called antipsychotics or neuroleptics. Most neuroleptics block D1 receptors but there is a close correlation between the clinical dose of antipsychotic drugs and their affinity for D2 receptors suggesting that blockade of this receptor subtype may be particularly important. D2 receptors occur in the limbic system, and in the basal ganglia, D3 and D4 receptors occur mainly in the limbic areas. It was hoped that selective antagonists at these receptors would provide antipsychotic drugs with fewer adverse motor effects but unfortunately they were ineffective.

Antipsychotic drugs require several weeks to control the symptoms of schizophrenia and most patients require maintenance treatment for many years. Relapses are common even in drug-maintained patients. Unfortunately, neuroleptics also block dopamine D2 receptors in the basal ganglia, often producing distressing and disabling movement disorders (e.g. parkinsonism, acute dystonic reactions, akathisia [motor restlessness] and tardive dyskinesia [orofacial and trunk movements] which may be irreversible; see Chapter 41). Blockade of D2 receptors in the pituitary gland causes an increase in prolactin release and endocrine effects (e.g. gynaecomastia, galactorrhoea; see Chapter 17). Many neuroleptics also block muscarinic receptors (causing dry mouth, blurred vision, constipation), α-adrenoceptors (postural hypotension) and histamine H1 receptors (sedation). Antipsychotic drugs have a wide variety of structures.

Phenothiazines

Chlorpromazine was the first phenothiazine used in schizophrenia and is still used although it produces more adverse effects than many newer drugs. It is very sedative and is particularly useful in violent patients.

Butyrophenones

Haloperidol is a potent drug with less sedative action and anticholinergic effects than chlorpromazine. However, it is associated with a high incidence of movement disorders.

Atypical drugs

Some newer drugs have a reduced tendency to cause movement disorders and are referred to as atypical agents (e.g. **clozapine**, **risperidone**, **olanzapine**, **quietiapine**). With the possible exception of clozapine, these drugs are not more efficacious than the older antipsychotic drugs. Clozapine is restricted to patients resistant to other drugs because it causes neutropenia or agranulocytosis in about 4% of patients. Risperidone and other newer atypical agents are increasingly used in the treatment of schizophrenia because they are more acceptable to patients.

It is not clear why some neuroleptics are 'atypical'. Clozapine may be atypical because in addition to be a dopamine D2 antagonist, it is a potent blocker of 5HT2 receptors. This idea is supported by an initial clinical trial in which ritanserin (a 5HT2 antagonist) apparently reduced the movement disorders caused by classic neuroleptics.

Depot preparations

Schizophrenic patients are, if possible, treated in the community. This has led to an increased use of long-acting depot injections for maintenance therapy. Oily injections of the decanoate derivatives of, for example, risperidone, may be given at intervals of 1–4 weeks.

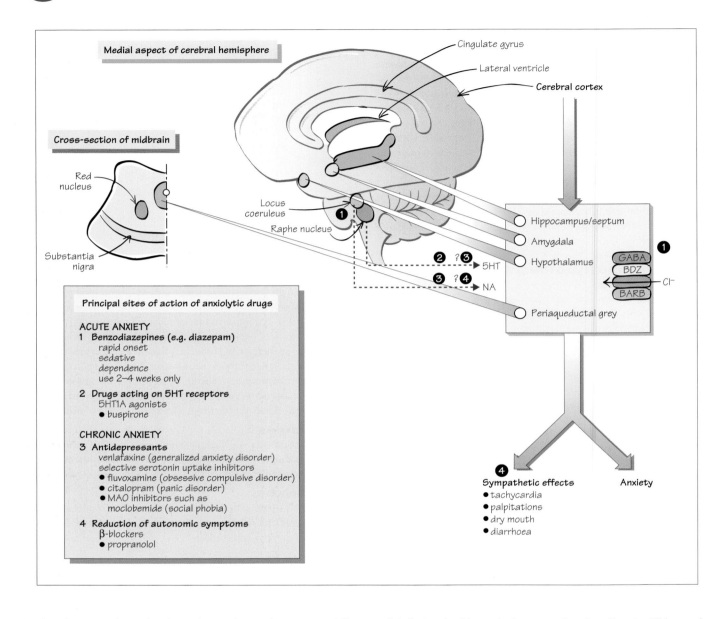

Anxiety is a normal emotional reaction to threatening or potentially threatening situations, and is accompanied by sympathetic overactivity. In **anxiety disorders** the patient experiences anxiety that is disproportionate to the stimulus, and sometimes in the absence of any obvious stimulus. There is no organic basis for anxiety disorders, the symptoms resulting from overactivity of the brain areas involved in 'normal' anxiety. Psychiatric disorders that occur without any known brain pathology are called **neuroses**.

Anxiety disorders are subdivided into four main types: ***generalized anxiety disorder***, ***panic disorder***, ***stress reactions*** and ***phobias***. Many transmitters seem to be involved in the neural mechanisms of anxiety, the evidence being especially strong for **γ-aminobutyric acid (GABA)** and **5-hydroxytryptamine (5HT)**. Because intravenous injections of **cholecystokinin (CCK₄)** into humans cause the symptoms of panic it has been suggested that abnormalities in different transmitter systems

might be involved in particular types of anxiety disorder. This remains to be seen.

The GABA-A receptor is affected by a cluster of genes on chromosome 5. However, there is no evidence for any chromosomal abnormality specifically linked with generalized anxiety disorder. There is some evidence for decreased GABA binding in the left temporal pole, an area concerned with experiencing and controlling fear and anxiety.

There may be disturbances of serotoninergic and noradrenergic transmission in anxiety. Thus, chlorophenylpiperazine (a non-specific 5HT1 and 5HT2 agonist) increased anxiety in patients with generalized anxiety disorder. These patients also show a reduced growth hormone response to clonidine (an α_2-receptor agonist) suggesting a decrease in α_2-receptor sensitivity. This response is also seen in patients with major depression. This is perhaps not surprising because genetic studies suggest that generalized anxiety disorder and major depression may have a common genetic basis and both disorders benefit from the administration of antidepressant drugs.

Treatment of mild anxiety disorders may only require simple *supportive psychotherapy*, but in severe anxiety anxiolytic drugs given for a short period are useful. The **benzodiazepines** (e.g. *diazepam*) produce their effects by enhancing GABA-mediated inhibition in many of the brain areas involved in anxiety, including the raphe nucleus. Some **antidepressants** (e.g. *amitriptyline, paroxetine*) have anxiolytic activity and they are used for the long-term treatment of anxiety disorders. Their mechanism of action in anxiety is unclear. β-**adrenoceptor antagonists** have a limited use in the treatment of situational anxiety (e.g. in musicians) where palpitations and tremor are the main symptoms. Efforts to discover non-sedative anxiolytics have led to the trial of several drugs that act on specific 5HT receptors but only one, *buspirone*, has been introduced.

Anxiety disorders

Generalized anxiety disorders have both psychological and physical symptoms. The psychological symptoms include a feeling of fearful anticipation, difficulty in concentrating, irritability and repetitive worrying thoughts that are often linked to awareness of sympathetic overactivity.

Phobic anxiety disorders have the same core symptoms as generalized anxiety disorders but occur only under certain circumstances, e.g. the appearance of a spider (arachnophobia). In contrast, *panic attacks* are episodic attacks of anxiety in which physical symptoms predominate (e.g. choking, palpitations, chest pain, sweating, trembling).

Benzodiazepines

Benzodiazepines (e.g. diazepam) are orally active central depressants but, in contrast to other hypnotics and anxiolytics, their maximum effect does not produce severe or fatal respiratory depression. They induce sleep when given in high doses at night (see Chapter 44) and provide sedation and reduce anxiety when given in divided doses during the day. They also have anticonvulsant activity (see Chapter 58), are muscle relaxants and produce amnesia. All these actions are brought about by the potentiation of the action of GABA on the GABA-A receptor which consists of five subunits. Variants of each of these subunits have been cloned (six α, three β and one γ). Several other subunits exist but it seems that most GABA-A receptors comprise two α_1, two β_2 and one γ_1 subunit. Benzodiazepines enhance the action of synaptically released GABA by binding to a benzodiazepine receptor site on the GABA-A receptor complex. This causes a conformational change to the GABA binding site, increasing its affinity for GABA. Studies in transgenic mice have shown that the α_1-subunit is required for sedative, hypnotic and anticonvulsant activity because a point mutation in this subunit renders the mice resistant to these actions (see also Chapter 44). In contrast, a mutation in the α_2-subunit results in mice that are resistant to the anxiolytic action of benzodiazepines.

The main adverse effects of the benzodiazepines are drowsiness, impaired alertness, agitation and ataxia. In anxiety disorders, benzodiazepines should only be given for a maximum of 2–3 weeks because longer treatment risks the development of **dependence**. If this occurs, stopping the drug frequently leads to a **withdrawal syndrome** characterized by anxiety, tremor, sweating and insomnia—symptoms similar to the original complaint.

Sites of action of benzodiazepines in the brain

The areas of the brain involved in the anxiolytic action of the benzodiazepines have been studied in rats by injecting tiny quantities of a drug through cannulae implanted in different brain areas. In general, limbic and brainstem structures seem important in mediating the anxiolytic actions of these drugs. In humans, cerebral blood flow and glucose metabolism studies using positron emission tomography (PET) have not revealed consistent differences in anxious and non-anxious subjects.

Buspirone

Serotonin (5HT) cell bodies are located in the raphe nuclei of the midbrain and project to many areas of the brain including those thought to be important in anxiety (hippocampus, amygdala, frontal cortex; see Chapter 54). In rats, lesions of the raphe nuclei produce anxiolytic effects, while stimulation of 5HT1A autoreceptors with agonists such as 8-hydroxy-DPAT produce anxiogenic effects. A role for 5HT in anxiety was strengthened when it was found that benzodiazepines reduce the turnover of 5HT in the brain and, when microinjected into the raphe nucleus, reduce the rate of neuronal firing and produce an anxiolytic effect. However, stimulation of postsynaptic 5HT1A receptors in limbic areas has anxiogenic effects. These opposing pre- and postsynaptic actions may explain why **buspirone**, a 5HT1A partial agonist, has limited efficacy and works after only several weeks. Specific antagonists at 5HT3 receptors (e.g. ondansetron) and 5HT2 receptors (e.g. ritanserin) have little, if any, anxiolytic actions in humans.

β-blockers

The evidence for the role of noradrenaline (norepinephrine) in anxiety is much less compelling than that for GABA and 5HT. Nevertheless, β-adrenoceptor antagonists (e.g. **propranolol**) have a limited use in the treatment of patients with mild or transient anxiety and where autonomic symptoms such as palpitations and tremor are the most troublesome symptoms. The beneficial effects of β-blockers in these patients may result from a peripheral action because those (e.g. practolol) that do not pass the blood–brain barrier are equally effective.

Peptides and anxiety

Several neuropeptides have been implicated in anxiety. The strongest evidence is for the anxiogenic effect of **corticotrophin-releasing hormone** (CRH), and CRH has also been implicated in depression. This raises the the theoretical possibility that a CRH receptor-1 antagonist may have anxiolytic actions and such drugs are under development. **Substance P** may also have anxiogenic effects and an NK1 receptor antagonist is in clinical trials for anxiety and depression. **CCK** is a gut peptide that also occurs in many areas of the brainstem and midbrain that are involved in emotion, mood and arousal. Because CCK4 is one of the few agents (CO_2 is another) that elicits genuine panic-like attacks, it was hoped that CCK antagonists would be useful anxiolytics. Unfortunately, clinical trials revealed that non-peptide CCK antagonists are ineffective in anxiety disorders.

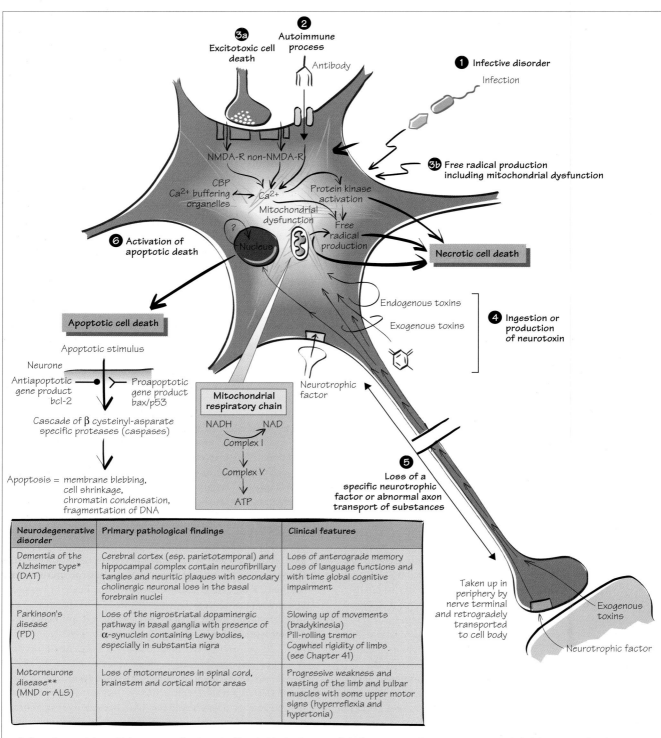

Neurodegenerative disorder	Primary pathological findings	Clinical features
Dementia of the Alzheimer type* (DAT)	Cerebral cortex (esp. parietotemporal) and hippocampal complex contain neurofibrillary tangles and neuritic plaques with secondary cholinergic neuronal loss in the basal forebrain nuclei	Loss of anterograde memory Loss of language functions and with time global cognitive impairment
Parkinson's disease (PD)	Loss of the nigrostriatal dopaminergic pathway in basal ganglia with presence of α-synuclein containing Lewy bodies, especially in substantia nigra	Slowing up of movements (bradykinesia) Pill-rolling tremor Cogwheel rigidity of limbs (see Chapter 41)
Motorneurone disease** (MND or ALS)	Loss of motorneurones in spinal cord, brainstem and cortical motor areas	Progressive weakness and wasting of the limb and bulbar muscles with some upper motor signs (hyperreflexia and hypertonia)

* Some forms of dementia have a more focal onset with selective involvement of the frontotemporal cortex, some cases of which have cortical inclusion (Pick) bodies at autopsy. These disorders are commonly termed frontotemporal dementia

** Motorneurone disease can present with either purely LMN or UMN features, but the most common presentation is with a combination of the two —a condition also known as amyotrophic lateral sclerosis (ALS)

NB A range of other neurodegenerative disorders are not discussed in this chapter and include Huntington's disease (Chapters 41 and 60) and spinocerebellar degenerations (Chapter 60). The mechanisms of cell death in these conditions may be similar to those described in this chapter

inflamed state. Thus, once triggered an immune response can be amplified and propagated by the elaboration of cytokines and induced MHC expression with the opening up of the BBB.

In these circumstances the **microglia** are thought to be important as the **antigen presenting cells** and their interaction with T-helper lymphocytes is then pivotal in generating a full-blown immunological reaction.

Clinical disorders of the central nervous system with an immunological basis

Multiple sclerosis (MS)

Multiple sclerosis is a common neurological disorder in which the patient characteristically presents with episodes of neurological dysfunction secondary to inflammatory lesions within the CNS. Pathologically, these lesions represent small areas of demyelination secondary to an underlying inflammatory (mainly T cell) infiltrate—the trigger and target for which is not clear. The lesions often resolve with remyelination and clinical recovery, although with time a permanent loss of myelin ensues with secondary axonal loss and the development of fixed disabilities.

To date the most successful therapies are high-dose intravenous methylprednisolone which hastens recovery from acute relapses but does not alter the long-term disease process, and β-interferon which reduces the relapse rate but again has, as yet, an unproven role in modifying the long-term prognosis. More aggressive immunotherapy with drugs such as CAMPATH may prove to be more effective, especially if given early on in the course of the disease.

Acute disseminated encephalomyelitis

This is a rare inflammatory demyelinating disease of the CNS that occurs as a complication of a number of infections and vaccinations (e.g. measles and rabies vaccination). It is a monophasic illness (unlike multiple sclerosis) characterized by widespread disseminated lesions throughout the CNS that pathologically consist of an intense perivascular infiltrate of lymphocytes and macrophages with demyelination. This condition resembles **experimental allergic encephalomyelitis** which is a well-characterized T-cell-mediated disorder against a component of myelin (probably myelin basic protein) induced by inoculating animals with a combination of sterile brain tissue and adjuvants. This disorder is often used experimentally to model MS.

Other immunological diseases

A number of other diseases with an immunological basis can affect the CNS and these include those diseases that primarily affect blood vessels (the **vasculitides**).

In addition, there is a rare group of disorders in which there is CNS dysfunction as a remote effect of a cancer, **paraneoplastic syndromes**. In these conditions antibodies to components of the CNS are generated, presumably triggered by the tumour, which then lead to neuronal cell death and the development of a neurological syndrome, e.g. anti-Purkinje cell antibodies cause a profound cerebellar syndrome by the immunological removal of this cell type in the cerebellum. The exact mechanism by which these antibodies exert their effect is not known as antibodies normally do not cross the BBB, but pathologically there is often evidence of a lymphocytic infiltrate in the affected structure which implies that the antibody is capable of inducing an immune-mediated process of neuronal loss.

Clinical disorders of the peripheral nervous system with an immunological basis

The PNS has fewer of the protective features of the CNS so is more susceptible to conventional immune-mediated diseases.

• The **peripheral nerve** is affected by a number of immunological processes, including **Guillain–Barré syndrome**. In this condition there is often a preceding illness (e.g. *Campylobacter jejuni* or cytomegalovirus infection) that induces an immune response which then cross-reacts with components in the peripheral nerve (e.g. certain gangliosides). This then induces focal demyelination in the peripheral nerve, which prevents it from conducting action potentials normally (see Chapter 6). In time the patient usually recovers although they may require immunotherapy with either plasma exchange or intravenous immunoglobulin. A similar condition is seen in some diseases where abnormal amounts of a component of antibodies are produced (the **paraproteinaemias**).

• The **neuromuscular junction** can be affected by immunological processes as occurs in **myasthenia gravis** and the **Lambert–Eaton myasthenic syndrome** (see Chapter 7).

• **Muscles** can be involved in inflammatory processes. The most common form of this is **polymyositis**, which is a T-cell-mediated condition associated with proximal weakness and pain. In contrast, **dermatomyositis** is a B-cell-mediated disease centred on blood vessels which causes a painful proximal muscle weakness in association with a florid skin rash. This latter condition can represent a paraneoplastic syndrome in more elderly patients with tumours in the lung, breast, colon or ovary.

60 Neurogenetic disorders

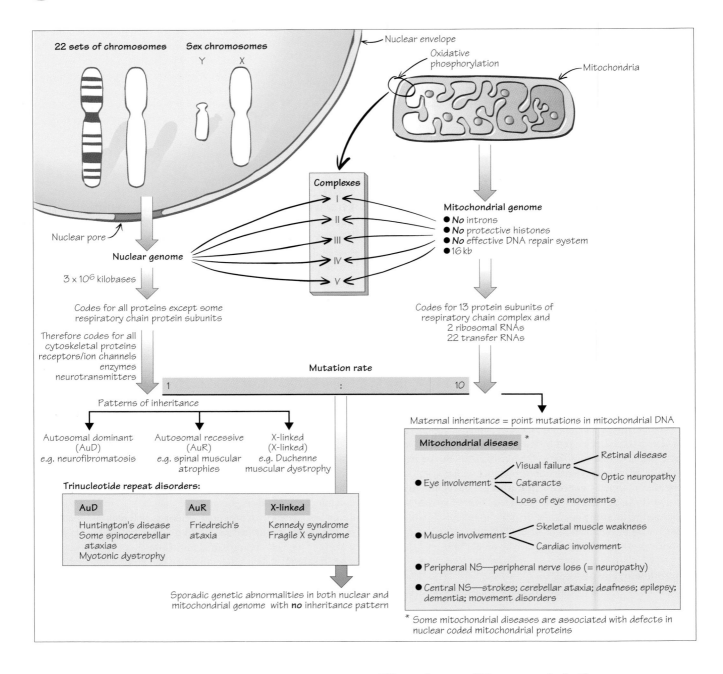

A large number of genetic disorders involve the nervous system, and some of these have pathology confined solely to this structure. Recent advances in molecular genetics have meant that many diseases of the nervous system are being redefined by their underlying genetic defect.

Two major new developments have revolutionized the role of genetic factors in the evolution of neurological disease. First, genes encoded in the maternally inherited **mitochondrial genome** can cause neurological disorders and, secondly, a number of inherited neurological disorders have as their basis an expanded trinucleotide repeat (**triplet repeat disorders**).

Disorders with gene deletions

Many different disorders within the nervous system result from the loss of a single gene or part thereof. For example, *hereditary neuropathy with a liability to pressure palsies*, in which the patient has a tendency to develop recurrent focal entrapment neuropathies in association with a large deletion on chromosome 17, which includes the gene coding for the peripheral myelin protein 22 (PMP 22).

Disorders with gene duplications

The duplication of a gene can, under some circumstances, cause disease. An example of this is in certain types of *hereditary motor and sensory neuropathy*, where the patient develops distal weakness, wasting and sensory loss in the first decades of life. In some of these cases there is duplication of part of chromosome 17, including the gene coding for PMP 22.

Disorders with gene mutations

This is the most common form of genetic defect and in these diseases there is a mutation in the gene coding for a specific enzyme or protein which results in that product failing to work normally.

An example of such a situation is found in some familial forms of *motorneurone disease* (see Chapter 57) and *muscular dystrophies* (see Chapter 10) as well as *myotonic syndromes* (see Chapter 5).

Disorders showing genetic imprinting

Genetic imprinting is the differential expression of autosomal genes depending upon their parental origin. Thus, disruption of the maternal gene(s) on a certain part of chromosome 15 (15q11-q13) causes *Prader–Willi syndrome* (mental retardation with obesity, hypogenitalism and short stature) while disruption of the same genes from the father causes *Angelman's syndrome* (a condition of severe mental retardation, cerebellar ataxia, epilepsy and craniofacial abnormalities).

Mitochondrial disorders

Mitochondria contain their own DNA and synthesize a number of the proteins in the respiratory chain responsible for oxidative phosphorylation (see Chapter 57), although the vast majority of mitochondrial proteins are encoded by nuclear DNA. Thus, mitochondrial disorders (deletions, duplication or point mutations) can result from defects in either these nuclear coded genes or the mitochondria genome. However, mitochondrial DNA mutates more than 10 times as frequently as nuclear DNA and has no introns (non-coding parts of the genome), so that a random mutation will usually strike a coding DNA sequence. As mitochondria are inherited from the fertilized oocyte, disorders with point mutations in the mitochondrially coded DNA show maternal inheritance (always inherited from the mother). However, within each cell there are many mitochondria and so a given cell can contain both normal and mutant mitochondrial DNA, a situation known as **hetero-plasmy** and it is only when a given threshold is reached that disease results.

The clinical disorders associated with different defects in the mitochondrial genome are legion, and the reason why some areas are targeted in some conditions and not others is not clear.

Trinucleotide repeat disorders

A number of different disorders have now been identified that have as their major genetic defect an expanded triplet repeat, i.e. there is a large and abnormal expansion of three bases in the genome. In normal individuals triplet repeat sequences are not uncommon but once the number of repeats exceeds a certain number the disease will definitely appear.

This pathological triplet (or trinucleotide) repeat either occurs in the coding part of a gene (e.g. *Huntington's disease*; see Chapter 41) or in a non-coding part of the genome (e.g. *Friedreich's ataxia*). The resulting expansion either causes a loss of function (e.g. frataxin in *Friedreich's ataxia*) or a new gain of function in that gene product (e.g. huntingtin in *Huntington's disease*). This latter aspect is of interest as the new protein appears to have a function that is unique to it and which is critical to the evolution of the neurodegenerative process. However, the mechanism by which this protein produces selective neuronal death in specific CNS sites is not known as many of the mutant gene products are widely expressed throughout the brain and body.

The consequence of a large unstable DNA sequence as occurs in these disorders is that the triplet repeat can increase during mitosis and meiosis, resulting in longer triplet repeat sequences (**dynamic mutations**). This means that the most likely time for triplet expansion is during spermatogenesis and subsequent fertilization/embryogenesis, and has two major implications. First, longer repeats tend to occur in the offspring of affected men and, secondly, longer repeats tend to occur in subsequent generations. This results in patients of subsequent generations presenting with earlier onset and more severe forms of the disorder—a phenomenon known as **genetic anticipation** as longer repeat sequences are associated with younger onset and more severe forms of the disease.

Case studies and questions

Case 1: A middle-aged woman with progressive weakness

You are called to see a 43-year-old woman in the accident and emergency department with a 5-day history of increasing weakness of all four limbs, lower back pain and sensory symptoms in her hands and feet. She has no significant previous medical or family history. She has recently been on holiday to the Canary Islands where she had a diarrhoeal illness.

On examination she has some slight facial weakness, a poor cough and weakness of the arms and legs, with no reflexes and a loss of feeling to light touch and pinprick to the wrist and ankle.

1 *What is the most likely diagnosis?*
2 *What test would you do to confirm this diagnosis?*
3 *What is the pathological basis of this disorder?*
4 *What might happen next in the course of this woman's illness?*
5 *Could this woman have myasthenia gravis, motorneurone disease or spinal cord compression given the back pain?*
6 *Is the information about her holiday relevant?*
7 *What treatment might you offer this woman?*

Case 2: A deaf young man with poor balance

A 28-year-old man reports increasing tinnitus in his right ear with a tendency to fall to the right. He has no significant previous medical history and on examination he has right-sided ataxia, a gaze paresis to the left and sensorineural deafness on that side.

1 *Where is the lesion?*
2 *What is the lesion likely to be?*
3 *Why does he have a gaze paresis?*
4 *Would you initially do a lumbar puncture in this man to help in the diagnosis?*
5 *What (other) tests would be helpful in the diagnosis of this man?*
6 *Should his family be told they are at risk of developing similar problems?*

Another patient with a similar story has severe pain in his ear with a history of chronic ear infection.

7 *Is there any other diagnosis you can think of in this patient?*
8 *What treatment should the patients have?*

Case 3: A case of progressive bulbar failure with double vision

A 65-year-old woman presents with a 3-month history of fatiguable double vision and dysphagia. She is a smoker of 10 cigarettes a day and has a previous medical history of thyroid disease which was treated with radioactive iodine and replacement thyroxine therapy. On examination she has restricted eye movements, bilateral ptosis and proximal limb weakness. Her forced vital capacity is 2.8 L. Her routine blood tests are normal. Her chest X-ray shows lower lobe collapse and pneumonia.

1 *Where is the pathology likely to be located in this woman?*
2 *What is the relevance of her previous medical history?*
3 *Are the smoking history and chest X-ray signs relevant?*
4 *What would help decide on the correct diagnosis?*
5 *The next day she seems better: why might this be the case?*
6 *Would steroid therapy help this woman?*

Case 4: Episodes of transient neurological dysfunction in an elderly man

A 72-year-old man presents with intermittent episodes of left-sided weakness involving his arm, face and leg. Each episode lasts about 20–30 minutes and they happen every day, 1–2 hours after getting up. He is hypertensive on medication (nifedipine—a Ca^{2+} channel antagonist) which he takes three times a day. He smokes 10 cigarettes a day. In the past he has had ischaemic heart disease and angina, and has pains in his calves when he walks about a quarter of a mile which go when he rests.

1 *What is wrong with his legs and should he have an urgent lumbar spine scan for this problem?*
2 *Which part of his nervous system is being affected in the left sided episode and what and where is the pathology likely to lie?*
3 *Why is speech not involved?*
4 *What would you look for on examination?*
5 *What investigations would you do?*
6 *Why do these attacks occur 2 hours after getting up?*
7 *What treatment would you offer this man?*

Case 5: Transient neurological dysfunction in a young woman

A 28-year-old woman presents with an episode of painful blurred vision in her left eye which comes on over a week and spontaneously recovers over an 8-week period. Six months later she presents with progressive leg weakness which has come on over 4 days with altered sensation in her legs. She has an aunt with Parkinson's disease.

On examination she has a nystagmus on left and right lateral gaze, a pale left optic disc on fundoscopy and some subtle but definite incoordination in the left arm. In the lower limbs she has a spastic left leg with loss of joint position sense and vibration perception threshold but reduced pinprick and temperature perception in the right leg to the level of T10.

1 *What was the problem with her eye and what field defect (if any) would you anticipate to find if you had seen her at the time of the original visual symptoms?*
2 *What is the syndrome affecting her legs?*
3 *Where is the lesion causing her leg symptoms?*
4 *Why is the sensory distribution different in the two legs?*
5 *What is the likely diagnosis and what is the underlying pathophysiological process?*
6 *Would scanning of the spine help in the diagnosis of this case?*

Case 6: A vegan with a progressive gait disorder

A 36-year-old vegan presents to his GP with progressive difficulty walking, numbness especially in the legs and some visual symptoms. He has an unstable, ataxic gait with spasticity in the legs, absent ankle jerks, reduced joint position sense and loss of light touch and pinprick to the wrists and ankles.

1 *Where is the pathology?*
2 *What could be causing his problem? Why and how would you prove this?*

3 *What other lesions or diseases can give spastic legs with absent ankle jerks?*

The MRI scan of his neck shows a lesion in the dorsal columns of the spinal cord.

4 *Could this account for his symptoms?*

Case 7: Slowing-up in a 60-year-old man

A 62-year-old man presents with a 6-month history of slowing up with a change in handwriting. His GP thinks he looks depressed and treats him with a selective serotonin reuptake inhibitor (SSRI) with no benefit. You are asked to see him to suggest another antidepressant. He has a previous medical history of Ménière's disease and has been on an antisickness tablet, metoclopramide, for this. His mother developed Alzheimer's disease in her eighties.

1 *What would you ask in the history of this patient?*
2 *What would you look for in your clinical examination?*
3 *What is the relevance of the previous medical and family history?*
4 *What would you do next in terms of investigation and management?*

Case 8: A young woman with a bad headache

A 22-year-old woman gives a 2-week history of headache with occasional loss of vision lasting a few seconds on standing or straining. On examination she has a body mass index of 33, bilateral papilloedema and no neurological deficits. Her computer tomography (CT) scan of her head is normal. She goes on to have a lumbar puncture which shows an opening pressure of 42 cm H_2O, 3 white cells, no red cells, 0.3 g/L protein and 3.2 mmol/L glucose.

1 *Is the cerebrospinal fluid normal and should any other tests have been carried out on it?*
2 *What are the two most likely diagnoses?*
3 *What further tests would you do to prove this?*
4 *What is the problem with her vision?*
5 *What treatment would you suggest?*
6 *What are the common causes of papilloedema?*

Case 9: Bulbar failure in a patient with history of cancer

A 58-year-old woman with a previous history of breast carcinoma presents with painful progressive dysphagia and dysarthria. On examination she has IXth, Xth and XIIth cranial nerve palsies. The CT scan of her brain is normal; her CSF shows 27 cells, 1.2 g/L protein and 1.1 mmol/L glucose with a serum glucose of 4.4 mmol/L.

1 *What is the most likely cause of her lower cranial nerve palsies?*
2 *How would you prove this diagnosis?*
3 *What is the prognosis?*
4 *Why was the CT scan unhelpful?*

Case 10: A young woman with evolving dizziness

A 21-year-old woman presents with a 2-week history of an evolving neurological problem consisting of dizziness, vomiting, oscillopsia, dysarthria and altered facial sensation. She has never had any previous illnesses and is on no treatment. On examination she has a complex eye movement disorder with nystagmus, ataxia bilaterally and a scanning dysarthria with some pyramidal signs in her legs. She also has some altered sensory feelings to light touch over the whole of her face.

1 *Where is the lesion?*

2 *What is the likely pathology of this lesion?*
3 *How would you prove this?*
4 *What treatment would you offer?*
5 *What is her prognosis?*

Case 11: Headache and weakness in a middle-aged patient

A 36-year-old woman presents with a 2-week history of increasing headache which is worse at night and in the early morning. Of late she has also become increasingly drowsy with an evolving left-sided hemiparesis. Her headache causes her to vomit and on occasions she has had involuntary movements of the left arm and leg and possibly of the face as well.

1 *Where is the lesion and why is she drowsy?*
2 *What is the cause of her involuntary movements of her left side?*
3 *What investigations would you organize and when relative to seeing the patient would you arrange for these to be carried out?*
4 *How would you prove your diagnosis?*

Case 12: An elderly woman who suddenly goes blind

A 74-year-old woman wakes up at night and asks her husband to turn on the lights. He informs her that they are already on. She went to bed perfectly fit and well.

1 *What is the problem?*
2 *What caused this problem?*
3 *What investigations would you organize?*

Case 13: A young man with neck pain, collapse and a quadriparesis

A 28-year-old man 'working out' in the gym suddenly develops severe neck pain and collapses to the ground. He cannot move his limbs and goes into respiratory arrest. He is resuscitated and moved to an intensive care unit where he is found to have normal cranial nerves but no movement of any limb. He is unable to breath on his own, has a loss of pinprick and temperature sensation to the shoulders but good preservation of joint position sense and vibration perception threshold.

1 *Where is the lesion?*
2 *What is the cause of the lesion?*
3 *Why has it happened?*
4 *What is the significance of the sensory loss?*

Case 14: An ever-increasingly painful foot in a young patient

An 18-year-old woman fractures her left ankle jumping off a horse. The ankle fracture repairs but soon afterwards she develops pain in her left foot. She has no significant previous medical history and on examination she has an exquisitely sensitive left foot and yells with pain when it is touched. The skin on the foot is shiny and flushed. Neurological examination of the foot is not possible but X-ray of the foot shows focal osteoporosis.

1 *What is the diagnosis?*
2 *What has caused it?*
3 *How would you treat it?*
4 *What would you not recommend for her to have?*

Case 15: An elderly man with a clumsy hand

A 64-year-old man presents with a 9-month history of a clumsy left arm and hand. He complains that he cannot control his left hand which tends to do its own thing. On examination he looks slightly parkinsonian with a stiff left arm and normal power with minimal sensory loss and normal coordination. However, when you ask him to do things with his left hand he is unable to do this.

1 *What is the most likely diagnosis?*
2 *Where might the lesion lie?*
3 *How would you prove the nature of the problem?*
4 *What rare condition may he have?*
5 *How would you treat the syndrome?*

Answers

Case 1: A middle-aged woman with progressive weakness

1 Guillain–Barré syndrome.

2 In the early stages of the disease the tests are often normal. However, nerve conduction studies should show evidence of slowing of nerve conduction as the condition is an acute demyelinating inflammatory neuropathy affecting all peripheral nerves as well as some of the cranial nerves.

3 This is normally an inflammatory response against components in the peripheral nerve and/or myelin, typically after some previous illness such as *Campylobacter jejuni* gastroenteritis or some viral infection. Thus, one sees inflammation in the nerve which leads to the stripping off of the myelin around the nerve; this gives the weakness and sensory loss as the nerve cannot conduct impulses normally.

4 It is possible that this woman will now plateau out with her clinical condition and slowly improve. However, there is a concern in someone with this degree of weakness that they will go on to develop worsening bulbar and respiratory failure. They should thus be managed on a high-dependency unit where their respiratory function can be assessed using forced vital capacity and they should probably be nil by mouth given the poor cough and risk of aspiration pneumonia. If her respiration were to get worse she would require ventilatory support. Also, a significant number of people with Guillain–Barré syndrome develop autonomic involvement and she could develop unstable blood pressures as well as possible cardiac arrhythmias; thus she should be monitored for this.

5 The information about the holiday may be relevant as many cases of Guillain–Barré syndrome have a preceding illness of which one of the most common is *Campylobacter jejuni* gastroenteritis. This can be tested for and it might well prove positive in this woman.

6 The treatment that should be offered to this woman, apart from the supportive therapy mentioned above, is some form of immunotherapy. This typically takes the form of either plasma exchange or intravenous immunoglobulin.

See Chapters 6, 8, 33, 43, 52 and 59.

Case 2: A deaf young man with poor balance

1 The lesion is clearly involving the right pons, right side of the brainstem or cerebellum and presumably the VIIIth cranial nerve on the right given the deafness. It is therefore likely that the lesion is in the cerebellar pontine angle on the right.

2 Given the position, the most likely cause of this is an acoustic neuroma, which is a schwannoma of the vestibular part of the VIIIth cranial nerve. There are a number of other lesions in this anatomical location that could give this clinical picture including meningiomas as well as different types of developmental cysts.

3 This reflects compression of the right pontine area, in particular the pontine paramedian reticular formation, which is responsible for horizontal gaze.

4 Definitely not. This patient clearly has some problem in the posterior fossa and no lumbar puncture should be undertaken in any patient with a lesion in this region of the neuro axis until imaging has been secured, and if a space occupying lesion is found, no lumbar puncture should be performed.

5 It is doubtful that any further tests are required outside a magnetic resonance imaging (MRI) scan. Sometimes, brainstem auditory evoked potentials can help detect abnormalities within the VIIIth cranial nerve to help localize the lesion but in this case it is unlikely to be helpful given that the patient is deaf.

6 No, as acoustic neuromas are rarely inherited. If they are bilateral in nature, however, this implies that the family might have a condition called neurofibromatosis type II in which case genetic testing and counselling would be advised.

7 Some patients develop malignant middle ear infections where the infection is such that it erodes the bone and destroys the local structures. In younger people this can take the form of cholesteatoma; in older patients—especially diabetics—it can often start in the external ear and patients develop a malignant otitis externa.

8 In the case of an acoustic neuroma the only treatment is a surgical removal of the lesion with sacrifice of the VIIIth cranial nerve. In the case of infection, clearly surgical and/or antibiotic therapy is required depending on the extent and nature of the lesion.

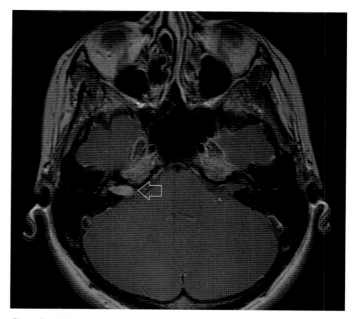

Case 2 MRI showing a small acoustic neuroma emerging from the internal auditory meatus.

See Chapters 13, 14, 28-30, 39, 42 and 52.

Case 3: A case of progressive bulbar failure with double vision

1 Given the extensive nature of the weakness involving the eye muscles, the eyelids and the proximal muscles it is almost certainly in the neuromuscular junction although it could possibly involve the nerve or muscle. The proximal limb weakness with involvement of the eyes would make myasthenia the most likely diagnosis.

2 Patients with a history of thyroid disease can develop thyroid eye disease in which they get restriction of eye movements and often bulging of the eyes, so-called exophthalmos. While she could have restricted eye movements as a consequence of a thyrotoxicosis and

thyroid disease, which could give her proximal weakness, it would not give her the bilateral ptosis.

3 Some patients can express the remote effects of cancer as a cause of their neurological problems—so-called paraneoplastic syndromes. However, myasthenia gravis is normally associated with thymomas and thus the history of smoking is probably not relevant in this case. While the chest X-ray may reveal an underlying cancer related to the smoking history it seems unlikely that this relates to her neurology as the Lambert–Eaton myasthenic syndrome that is associated with lung cancer does not cause a restriction of eye movements. The more likely explanation of her chest X-ray signs is that she has had an aspiration pneumonia as a result of her palatal weakness and dysphagia.

4 The diagnosis of myasthenia gravis can be achieved using blood tests looking for anti-acetylcholine receptor and muscle-specific kinase (MUSK) antibodies. Neurophysiology will reveal deficits at the neuromuscular junction and one can go on to perform a Tensilon test where one gives a short-acting acetylcholinesterase inhibitor which enhances transmission at the neuromuscular junction and will transiently improve her neurology if she does have myasthenia gravis.

5 Myasthenia gravis causes fatigable weakness and often patients report worsening symptoms as the day goes on and as the muscles get used. This might account for why she is better the next day.

6 The typical management of patients with myasthenia gravis is to improve transmission at the neuromuscular junction using oral acetylcholinesterase inhibitors. However, the underlying condition is an immunological one and thus patients require immunosuppressive therapy. Typically, this is done orally with steroids along with other agents such as azathioprine. It is always recommended that steroids are started at low dose as paradoxically patients with myasthenia gravis can get much worse initially with high-dose steroid medication, although the evidence that this is truly the case with myasthenia and steroid therapy is debatable.

See Chapters 7, 13, 14, 42, 52 and 59.

Case 4: Episodes of transient neurological dysfunction in an elderly man

1 The most likely explanation for the pain in his legs is intermittent claudication caused by restricted blood flow as a result of atherosclerotic change in the main arteries to the legs. It is very unlikely that a lumbar spine scan would help although some patients develop lumbar canal stenosis as a result of degenerative change in the lumbar spine. Typically, these patients develop exercise-induced back pain and sensory symptoms in their legs with pain and weakness.

2 In order for him to develop symptoms involving the whole of the left side of his body the lesion must lie above the level of the brainstem in the right hemisphere. Given the intermittent nature of the symptoms and their sudden onset it is likely to be vascular in nature, and given his history of hypertension and smoking in a man of this age the pathology is likely to lie within his carotid artery on the right causing him to have intermittent ischaemia of the right hemisphere in the distribution of the middle cerebral artery.

3 Speech is typically localized in the left hemisphere because this is the dominant hemisphere. Even in people who are left-handed the majority still have speech localized to the left hemisphere.

4 The main things to look for on the examination would be any residual neurology down the left side—in particular whether he has any weakness and numbness as well as looking for abnormalities in the right carotid artery such as a bruit. It would also be important to carry out a full cardiovascular examination to assess the health of his other arteries as well as his heart.

5 The standard investigations for people who have transient ischaemia of this nature is to image the carotid artery on that side with either an ultrasound scan or some form of MRI. In addition, one would probably wish to image his brain to see the extent to which he has ischaemic damage there. One would also look for further risk factors for cardiovascular disease such as fasting serum levels of cholesterol and glucose, as well as investigations of his heart (electrocardiogram, echocardiogram, etc.) if this has not been carried out already.

6 The explanation for this is that his blood pressure probably drops as a consequence of taking his antihypertension treatment. The drop in blood pressure is such that, combined with the carotid stenosis on that side, he has underperfusion of his right hemisphere giving him the symptoms that he describes. Thus, a change in antihypertensive medication to a slow-release, longer-acting treatment or milder agent may alleviate the attacks that he is describing.

7 Apart from the possible change in his antihypertensive treatment the management would depend on the degree of stenosis within the carotid artery. If this is less than 50–70% one would typically manage him medically with antiplatelet therapy such as aspirin as well as treat-

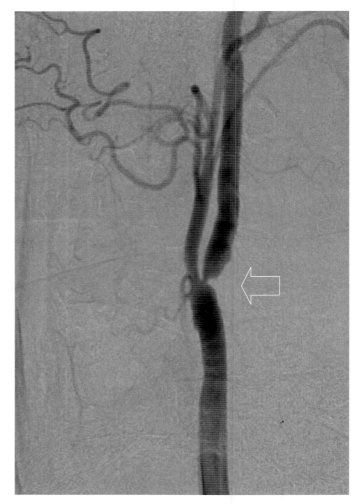

Case 4 Carotid angiogram showing a tight stenosis at the origin of the internal carotid artery, with a normal external and common carotid artery.

ments for any diabetes or hypercholesterolaemia if these are found to be present. If the stenosis is greater than 70% then he would probably be offered a surgical correction of his carotid stenosis with a carotid endarterectomy. He should also be told to stop smoking.
See Chapters 19, 34, 43, 52 and 53

Case 5: Transient neurological dysfunction in a young woman

1 The most likely diagnosis in this woman is multiple sclerosis given the distribution of neurology over time and space in someone of this age. The initial problem therefore was likely to be one of optic neuritis or inflammation within the left optic nerve. The characteristic visual field defect one sees in patients in the acute stages of optic neuritis are involvement of the central field with a scotoma.

2 This woman clearly has Brown–Séquard syndrome in that she has spasticity of the left leg with loss of dorsal column sensory loss on that side but spinothalamic sensory loss in the right leg.

3 The lesion must lie in the left side of the spinal cord above the level of T10.

4 On the ipsilateral side she has loss of the dorsal columns that project up ipsilaterally to the dorsal column nuclei in the lower medulla before crossing over to form the medial lemniscus. In contrast, the spinothalamic tract input (which conveys pain and temperature) crosses on entering the spinal cord and thus passes up contralateral to the side of entry.

5 The most likely diagnosis in this woman is multiple sclerosis as she has two neurological episodes separated in space and time involving sites that are preferentially involved in this disease process. The pathophysiological process is inflammatory demyelinating disease of the central nervous system.

6 Scanning of the spine would inform you as to whether she has inflammatory lesions in the spinal cord, which is important as there is

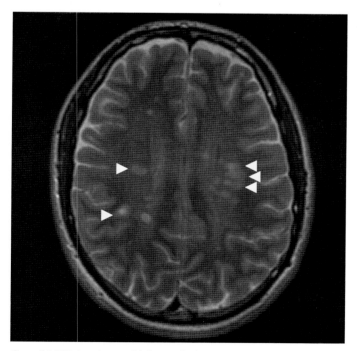

Case 5 MRI showing multiple small plaques of inflammation/demyelination characteristic of MS.

an outside possibility that she has some other cause for her Brown–Séquard syndrome such as a compressive spinal cord lesion. However, this seems very unlikely given her age, the absence of pain and the previous history of optic neuritis. The diagnosis of multiple sclerosis is made based on the history and examination, MRI scanning showing inflammatory lesions, and cerebrospinal fluid (CSF) examination showing evidence of intrathecal immunoglobulin production and in some cases evoked potentials typically involving the visual pathway to show that there has been previous episodes of demyelination within that pathway with consequent slowing of nerve conduction from the retina to the visual cortex.
See Chapters 12, 13, 33, 42, 43, 52, 53 and 59.

Case 6: A vegan with a progressive gait disorder

1 It is difficult in this man to be certain of the site of the pathology as he clearly has evidence of peripheral nerve involvement with absent ankle jerks and sensory loss in a glove and stocking distribution in his hands and feet. However, this cannot account for his spasticity as this would imply an upper motorneurone lesion and therefore involvement of the central nervous system. The ataxia could conceivably be brought about by his peripheral neuropathy although of course there could be a central component for it. Therefore, the most likely pathological process in this man involves both his central and peripheral nervous system.

2 In someone who is a vegan, the most likely explanation with peripheral and central nervous system involvement, is vitamin B_{12} deficiency. This can be easily proven by simply measuring serum B_{12} levels. B_{12} is necessary for the myelination of both peripheral and central nerves.

3 Clearly anything that involves the peripheral and central nervous system motor pathways could do this, such as motorneurone disease. Rare causes are some forms of leucodystrophies but it is always important to remember that a lesion in the lower part of the spinal cord in the region of the conus can give this syndrome. Finally, it is possible to have two different pathologies such as lumbar disc disease causing the loss of ankle jerks and an independent spinal cord lesion or compression causing the spastic legs such as a cervical myelopathy from cervical degenerative disease.

4 Yes, as it could reflect demyelination in his dorsal columns as a result of his B_{12} deficiency. However, it could not account for all of his symptoms given that he also has a glove and stocking sensory loss which would be most unusual for a lesion in this site. This latter symptom is more likely to reflect peripheral nerve demyelination secondary to the B_{12} deficiency.
See Chapters 12, 22, 33, 34–36, 43, 52 and 53.

Case 7: Slowing-up in a 60-year-old man

1 The most likely diagnosis in this patient is some form of parkinsonian syndrome. This may have been provoked by the use of antiemetic medication, some of which block the dopamine receptors, and this includes metoclopramide. Thus, it is important in this patient to find out whether his symptoms came on with the treatment for his Ménière's disease. If one suspects Parkinson's disease then it is useful to find out whether he has developed an asymmetric rest tremor; a change in his handwriting such that it has become smaller; a voice that has become quieter; and whether he has noticed that he does not swing one of his arms and walks with a slight dragging of one leg, and has slowed up in general.

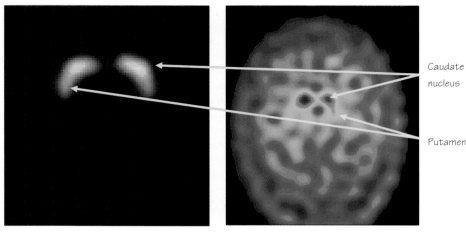

NORMAL   PARKINSON'S DISEASE

Caudate nucleus

Putamen

Case 7 A DaT scan showing loss of dopamine transporter signal, more in the putamen than candate in a patient with Parkinson's disease.

2 Given that one suspects this man has Parkinson's disease one would look for an absence of facial expression, so-called hypomimia, and a quiet voice, hypophonia. His eye movements may reveal some hypometric saccades. In the limbs he may have increased tone of a cogwheel nature with a resting tremor and bradykinesia. This is typically mainly or only down one side in early disease. On walking he may have a stooped gait with an absence of arm swing and a degree of shuffling, and some problems turning, with some postural instability.

3 The family history is almost certainly irrelevant given that a significant number of people will develop Alzheimer's disease in their ninth decade. The previous medical history is only relevant in so much as the patient may have been put on a dopamine-blocking antiemetic that has provoked their parkinsonian syndrome.

4 The investigation of Parkinson's disease often relies on the ruling out of other conditions. The vast majority of people rely on history and clinical examination for the diagnosis. Dopamine imaging is now available and this can be carried out to see whether there is dopamine deficiency within the striatum. The easiest way to do this is through a dopamine marker, such as dopamine transporter (DaT) scan in the nuclear medicine department. Management would depend on the extent to which the patient is incapacitated by their symptoms. In the first instance one would stop the antiemetic and review the patient. If they still have symptoms and require treatment then traditionally one would use dopamine replacement therapy in the form of dopamine agonists or levodopa.

See Chapters 34, 40, 41, 42, 43, 51, 52, 53 and 57.

Case 8: A young woman with a bad headache

1 The CSF, in terms of its constituents, is normal although one clearly needs to make sure that her serum glucose is taken such that the CSF is still approximately half that of the serum. The most striking abnormality in this woman is the markedly raised opening pressure as this should be less than 20 cm H_2O.

2 The most likely diagnoses in a woman of this age with a normal brain scan and this body mass index along with papilloedema and raised opening pressure is either benign intracranial hypertension or raised pressure caused by a sagittal sinus thrombosis.

3 In order to exclude a major venous sinus thrombosis or obstruction as a cause of her symptoms she requires imaging of her venous sinuses which is typically carried out using magnetic resonance venography (MRV). One can go on to do formal angiography if the MRV is equivocal.

4 The phenomenon that she is describing is visual obscuration. This is as a result of the transient rises in her CSF pressure which is greater than her arterial blood pressure giving her transient ischaemia of the optic nerve head. If this were to continue then there is a real risk that she will infarct her optic nerve head and she will become blind.

5 This depends on the aetiological cause. If she has a sagittal sinus thrombosis, she needs investigation to make sure she does not have

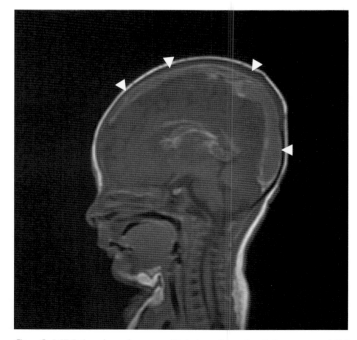

Case 8 MRI showing a large sagittal sinus thrombosis in a young child (***not*** a young adult as in the case history given)

some underlying coagulopathy and treatment with anticoagulants, typically warfarin, for 6 months. If she has normal sagittal sinuses and the diagnosis is benign intracranial hypertension then while the condition is benign, it can lead to irreversible visual loss and blindness for the reasons given above. Typically, the management involves losing weight and the use of acetazolamide as a way of reducing the production of CSF. If this fails to improve the situation more radical approaches are possible including shunting to reduce the CSF pressure. This is typically performed with a lumboperitoneal shunt.

6 The common causes of papilloedema is raised intracranial pressure. This is typically caused by mass lesions but can be a result of raised pressure as a consequence of benign intracranial hypertension as well as sagittal sinus thrombosis. It is also seen with malignant hypertension and a range of other rare causes. However, when present, the blood pressure needs to be checked and urgent imaging organized. Only if these are normal should a lumbar puncture be undertaken.

See Chapters 18, 19, 52 and 53.

Case 9: Bulbar failure in a patient with history of cancer

1 The most likely diagnosis in this case is malignant meningitis. This involves the seeding of the tumour on the meninges where it grows and in the process of which it picks off nerves, typically the lower lumbar and cranial nerves. It is often painful and so the constellation of progressive lower cranial nerve palsies with pain in a woman with previous breast carcinoma would make this the most likely diagnosis. Furthermore, the CSF examination is very much in keeping with malignat meningitis given the high number of cells, raised protein and low glucose.

2 While tuberculous meningitis is a possibility, the way to prove the diagnosis would be to perform cytology on the specimen of CSF to see whether the cells within it look like breast carcinoma cells. In order to exclude tuberculosis one would have to do specific stains and PCR to look for the infective organism.

3 The prognosis for malignant meningitis is often extremely poor although there are rare cases of people responding to chemotherapy and in the case of breast carcinoma, drugs that target the oestrogen receptor may be helpful such as tamoxifen. Generally speaking, the

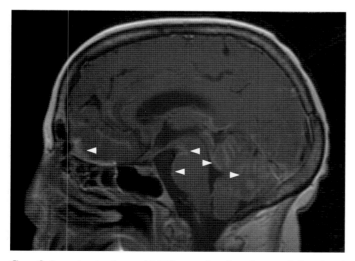

Case 9 A contrast enhanced MRI scan showing abnormal signal and thickening of meninges.

disease progresses rapidly with most patients dying within a few months of onset.

4 The CT scan was unhelpful in so much as it is very poor at looking at the meninges as well as the posterior fossa, however it was helpful at excluding a mass lesion in the brainstem. Quite often the diagnosis of malignant meningitis can be difficult as the meninges are involved in a disseminated fashion with relatively little in the way of thickening, and even on an MRI scan with contrast one often cannot see any abnormalities on the scan.

See Chapters: 13, 14, 18, 52 and 53.

Case 10: A young woman with evolving dizziness

1 The most likely site for this lesion is somewhere in the posterior fossa, probably involving the brainstem given the constellation of abnormalities as described. In order to get a complex eye movement disorder the lesion must involve the pons or the midbrain and this could also account for some of the ataxia although there may be spread of the lesion into the cerebellar peduncles. The altered sensation over the face would again point towards a brainstem lesion, this time slightly higher given that the whole face is involved and thus the lesion must reside somewhere in the upper midbrain.

2 The most likely pathology of this lesion is an inflammatory demyelinating plaque characteristic of multiple sclerosis given her age, the evolving presentation over 2 weeks and the absence of any previous medical history. It is possible that it could be a space occupying lesion or some other infective cause but this seems very unlikely given the nature of the progression and the relatively high prevalence of multiple sclerosis in the population.

3 In order to prove this as a diagnosis one would have to arrange for her to have an MRI scan to look at the nature of the abnormality in the brainstem with a view to going on to a lumbar puncture looking specifically for evidence of inflammation typically in the form of oligoclonal bands in the CSF but not the serum. One can also look for disseminated lesions in other sites typically within the visual pathway using visual evoked responses.

4 The treatment you would offer to some extent depends on the nature of the disability. However, brainstem problems are often very debilitating and while one can give symptomatic treatment such as antiemetics this woman probably merits a course of steroids to try and speed up the natural recovery that is characteristic of lesions of this type.

5 The prognosis is that she should make a good recovery from this lesion but that it is likely that she will go on to have further episodes and progressive disability, which may lead to consideration of disease modifying therapy targeting specific aspects of the immune system.

See Chapters 12, 13, 33, 42, 43, 52, 53 and 59.

Case 11: Headache and weakness in a middle-aged patient

1 The most likely site of this lesion given the left-sided hemiparesis is something in the right hemisphere. It is possible it could involve the right brainstem or upper cervical cord but involvement of the face with involuntary movement would exclude the cervical cord and brainstem lesions causing a pure hemiparesis would be unusual. The drowsiness relates to the increased intracranial pressure for which she has the classic story with early morning headache, vomiting and nausea along with the evolving drowsiness.

2 The cause of involuntary movements of her left side are almost certainly small epileptic seizures, in other words simple partial seizures of a motor type.

3 The investigation that needs to be carried out urgently is a CT scan as she has symptoms of raised intracranial pressure which could also be confirmed by looking for papilloedema on fundoscopy. This needs to be performed urgently given her evolution and the nature of her symptoms.

4 In order to prove the diagnosis one would need to perform a biopsy although quite often the imaging abnormalities coupled to the history are suggestive of primary gliomas. Importantly, secondary cancer deposits (with a primary tumour located at another site in the body) in the brain are common and thus searching for a tumour at another site may be needed. However, in order to prove beyond doubt that the tumour is what you think it is a biopsy is necessary.

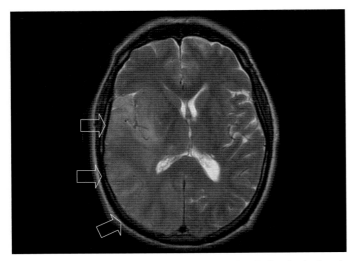

Case 11 MRI showing a diffuse space occupying lesion in the hemisphere, characteristic of a glioma.

See Chapters 4, 15, 18, 34, 51, 52, 53 and 58.

Case 12: An elderly woman who suddenly goes blind

1 This woman has clearly developed bilateral blindness. This is very unlikely to involve the eyes themselves as it would require a simultaneous bilateral anterior ischaemic optic neuropathy with complete visual loss. Thus, it is much more likely that the lesion resides within her occipital lobe and that she has had a bilateral occipital infarct from a lesion at the top of the basilar artery with involvement of both posterior cerebral arteries.

2 The cause of the problem is that she either has had an embolus pass up the basilar artery from her heart (or rarely a dissected vertebral artery) or less likely that she has atheromatous disease there and has occluded her vascular system as a consequence of thrombosis *in situ*.

3 The investigations that you organize would be an urgent scan to see the extent to which your diagnosis is right. However, in the acute stage infarcts can often be hard to see on CT or MRI scan. If an infarct is confirmed then one would look for the cardiovascular risk factors associated with stroke such as diabetes, high cholesterol or hypertension. One would also look for an embolic source for her stroke and this would involve ECG recordings from the heart, a 24-hour ECG from the heart

and an echocardiogram. If one is confident the stroke is very recent (less than 4 hours ago), one may consider thrombolytic therapy.
See Chapters 19, 26, 27, 33, 52 and 53.

Case 13: A young man with neck pain, collapse and a quadriparesis

1 The site of the lesion given the sensory level and the involvement of all four limbs is the upper cervical cord above C4 given that he is unable to breath. It cannot involve the brainstem given the absence of any cranial nerve signs.

2 The likely cause of the lesion is a vascular one given the acute onset and with the dissociated sensory loss, it implies that he has had an anterior spinal artery occlusion.

3 It is well described in some people 'working out' in gyms that they can have a fibrocartilaginous embolus in the anterior spinal artery. The occlusion of the anterior spinal artery in the cervical cord will lead to infarction of the anterior two-thirds of the spinal cord resulting in a flaccid quadraparesis in the first instance with sensory loss to pinprick and temperature and relative preservation of dorsal column function, namely joint position sense and vibration.

4 The significance of the sensory loss is that this is very characteristic of anterior spinal artery occlusion.
See Chapters 12, 19, 33, 43, 51, 52 and 53.

Case 14: An ever-increasingly painful foot in a young patient

1 The most likely diagnosis is one of reflex sympathetic dystrophy, now renamed complex regional pain syndrome. This is likely to be the case given the injury leading on to the exquisitely painful foot with evidence of autonomic dysfunction as seen with the flushed shiny skin and osteoporosis.

2 The cause of this is largely unknown but is well described in the context of relatively minor injuries, and may have an explanation in the abnormal expression of adrenoreceptors on peripheral nociceptors.

3 The treatment of this is often complicated but emphasis is put on trying to deal with the sympathetic nervous system through local sympathectomies.

4 The important thing is to try to treat her symptoms using a range of local measures and painkillers and she should resist the temptation to have an amputation or some other nerve lesion treatment as a way of trying to deal with her problems, as this often greatly aggravates the situation and can lead to phantom limb pain.
See Chapters 23 and 24.

Case 15: An elderly man with a clumsy hand

1 The diagnosis is clearly difficult as he appears to have normal sensation and power in the hand but is unable to use it. Thus, the differential diagnosis lies between some form of functional non-neurological psychiatric disorder or more likely dyspraxia. Dyspraxia is a term used to describe the inability to coordinate movements in the absence of overt motor and sensory deficits.

2 The most likely site for the lesion is the posterior parietal cortex in the right hemisphere.

3 The way in which one could prove the nature of the problem is to get the patient to carry out actions such as saluting, combing his hair, stirring a cup of tea as well as copying meaningless gestures that you do with your own hand. He will probably have an inability to do these,

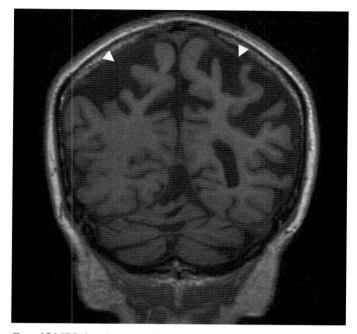

Case 15 MRI showing marked atrophy bilaterally in the region of the posterior parietal cortex.

thus confirming the diagnosis of dyspraxia. A scan would also help if it confirmed pathology in the right posterior parietal cortex.

4 The rare condition that he may have is corticobasal degeneration which is a progressive neurodegenerative disorder that has pathology around the central sulcus and deep within the basal ganglia. Typically, patients present with a parkinsonian syndrome with marked dyspraxia and asymmetry of deficits.

5 Unfortunately there is no way of treating this syndrome as it is refractory to all known medications.

See Chapters 15, 32, 33, 34, 43, 52, 53 and 57.

Appendix 1: Major neurotransmitter types

Neurotransmitter	Distribution	Receptor types	Associated neurological disorders
Amino acids			
Excitatory			
Glutamate	Widespread throughout CNS	1. Ionotropic: Non-NMDA (AMPA; kainate; quisqualate receptors) NMDA 2. Metabotropic	Epilepsy (Ch 58) Excitotoxic cell death (Ch 57)
Inhibitory			
GABA	Widespread throughout CNS	GABA-A GABA-B	Spinal cord motor disorders (Ch 36) Epilepsy (Ch 58) Anxiety (Ch 56)
Glycine	Spinal cord	Glycine	Startle syndromes (Ch 36)
Monoamines*			
Noradrenaline (nor-epinephrine)	Locus coeruleus to whole CNS (Ch 13) Postganglionic sympathetic nervous system (Ch 16)	$\alpha 1$; $\alpha 2$ $\beta 1$; $\beta 2$	Depression (Ch 54) Autonomic failure (Ch 16)
Serotonin (5-hydroxytryptamine)	Raphe nucleus in brainstem to whole CNS (Ch 55)	5HT1 (A–F) 5HT2 (A–C) 5HT3–5–HT7	Depression (Ch 54) Anxiety (Ch 56) Migraine
Dopamine	Nigrostriatal pathway in basal ganglia (Ch 40) Mesolimbic and mesocortical pathways (Chs 48 and 55) Retina (Ch 25) Hypothalamic–pituitary projection (Ch 17)	D1–D5 receptors on activation cause an increase in intracellular cAMP D2 receptors cause a decrease in intracellular cAMP on activation D3–D4 are independent of cAMP signalling system	Parkinson's disease (Ch 41) Schizophrenia (Ch 55) Control of pituitary hormone secretion (Ch 17) Control of vomiting Drug addiction (Ch 48)
Acetylcholine	Neuromuscular junction (Ch 7) Autonomic nervous system (Ch 16) Basal forebrain to cerebral cortex and limbic system (Ch 46, 57) Interneurones in many CNS structures including striatum (Ch 40)	Nicotinic Muscarinic (M1–M3 subtypes)	Disorders of the neuromuscular junction (Ch 7) Autonomic failure (Ch 16) Dementia of the Alzheimer type (Ch 57) Parkinson's disease (Ch 41) Epilepsy (Ch 58) Sleep–wake cycle (Ch 44)
Neuropeptides	Widespread distribution in CNS but especially are found in: dorsal horn of spinal cord (Ch 23, 24) basal ganglia (Ch 40) autonomic nervous system (Ch 16)	Various	See: Pain systems (Ch 23, 24) Basal ganglia (Ch 40) Autonomic nervous system (Ch 16) Neural plasticity (Ch 50) Anxiety (Ch 56) Sleep (Ch 44)
Others Purinergic ATP Endozapines			

*Histamine and adrenaline (noradrenaline) are monoamines that are found primarily in the hypothalamus and adrenal medulla, respectively.

Appendix 2a: Ascending sensory pathways in the spinal cord

Tract	Spinothalamic tract (STT)	Dorsal column–medial lemniscal pathway	Spinocerebellar tract (SCT)
Relevant chapter	23	22	39
Site of origin	Dorsal horn (Laminae I, III, IV and V) Crosses midline in spinal cord	Primary afferents from mechanoreceptors, muscle and joint receptors	Spinal cord interneurones and proprioceptive information from muscle and joint
Termination	Somatotopic organization with more caudal fibres added laterally Projects to brainstem and contralateral thalamus	Somatotopic organization with fibres terminating in dorsal column nuclei of medulla Decussate at this level to form medial lemniscus that synapses in ventroposterior nucleus of the thalamus	Two tracts: Dorsal SCT relays information from muscle and joint receptors via inferior cerebellar peduncle to cerebellum Ventral SCT relays information from spinal cord interneurons via superior cerebellar peduncle to cerebellum
Function	Conveys pain and temperature	Conveys proprioception, light touch and vibration	Conveys proprioceptive information as well as information of on-going activity in spinal cord interneurones

Appendix 2b: Descending motor tracts

Tract	Corticospinal or pyramidal tract (CoST)	Rubrospinal tract (RuST)	Vestibulospinal tract (VeST)	Reticulospinal tract (ReST)
Relevant chapters	34, 36–38	34, 36, 39	34, 36, 39	34, 36, 39
Site of origin	Primary motor cortex (40%) Premotor cortex (30%) Somatosensory cortex (30%)	Magnocellular part of red nucleus in midbrain	Deiter's nucleus in the medulla (part of the vestibular nuclear complex)	Caudal reticular formation in pons and medulla
Major actions	Important in independent fractionated finger movements A role in sensory processing (see Ch 22)	Projects to a similar population of MNs as CoST, namely those concerned with distal motor control Experimentally lesions of this tract produce little deficit unless combined with lesions of the CoST Its existence and significance in humans is debated	Innervates predominantly the extensor and axial muscles, and as such is important in the control of posture and balance	The ReST has both an excitatory and inhibitory input to the spinal cord interneurones and to a lesser extent MNs This pathway is important in damping down activity within the spinal cord such that a loss of this pathway produces profound extensor tone

The tectospinal tract is a relatively minor tract originating from the tectum in the midbrain. It is briefly discussed in Chapters 26, 34 and 36.

Appendix 3: Functional and anatomical systems of the cerebellum

System	SpinoCBM or paleoCBM: vermal region	SpinoCBM or paleoCBM: paravermal or intermediate region	PontoCBM or neoCBM	VestibuloCBM or ArcheoCBM
Major afferent connections	Vestibular nucleus Proximal limb Ia/Ib afferents and interneuronal activity relayed via DSCT and VSCT respectively Visual and auditory information to posterior lobe only	Ia/Ib afferents from distal limb via DSCT Interneuronal activity from distal spinal motor pools relayed in VSCT Primary motor and somatosensory cortex	Posterior parietal cortex Primary and premotor motor cortical area *Both* relayed via pontine nuclei	Semicircular canals via vestibular nucleus Visual information from superior colliculus, lateral geniculate nucleus and primary visual cortex relayed via pontine nuclei
Associated deep cerebellar nucleus	Fastigial	Interpositus (globose and emboliform)	Dentate	—
Major efferent projections	Reticular formation → ReST Vestibular nucleus → VeST (ventromedial descending motor pathways)	Red nucleus (magnocellular part) → RuST VA–VL nucleus of the thalamus → PMC (Brodmann's area 6) and MsI (Brodmann's area 4) → corticospinal tract (Dorsolateral descending motor pathways)	VA–VL nucleus of thalamus → Area 4 and 6 → corticospinal tract Red nucleus (parvocellular part) → inferior olive → CBM (Mollaret's triangle)	Vestibular nucleus → VeST Vestibular nucleus → oculomotor nuclei
Specific role	Control of axial musculature Regulate muscle tone	Distal limb coordination Regulate muscle tone	Motor planning Visual control of movement Minor role in distal limb coordination	Posture Eye movement control

Colour shading at the top of the table refers to Chapter 39.

Appendix 4: References

Chapter 2
Chizhikov VV and Millen KJ (2004) Mechanisms of roof plate formation in the vertebrate CNS. *Nature Neuroscience Reviews* **5**:808–812.

Chapter 6
Bean BP (2007) The action potential in mammalian central neurons. *Nature Neuroscience Reviews* **8**:451–465.

Chapter 23 and 24
Flor H, Nikolajsen L, Jensen TS (2006) Phantom Limb pain: a case of maladaptive CNS plasticity? *Nature Neuroscience Reviews* **7**: 873–881.

Chapter 25
Solomon SG and Lennie P (2007) The machinery of colour vision. *Nature Neuroscience Reviews* **8**:276–286.

Chapter 26
Lockley SW, Gooley JJ (2006) Circadian photoreception: Spotlight on the brain. *Curr.Biology* **16**:R795–797.

Chapter 28
Fettiplace R and Hackney CM (2006) The sensory and motor roles of auditory hair cells.*Nature Neuroscience Reviews* **7**:19–29.
LeMasurier M, Gillespie PG (2007) Hair bundles:keeping it together. *Nature Neurosci.* **10**:11–12.

Chapter 30
Day BL and Fitzpatrick RC (2005). The vestibular system. *Current Biology* **15**:R583–586.

Chapter 31
Simon SA, de Araujo IE, Gutierrez R, Nicolelis MAL (2006) The neural mechanisms of gustation: a distributed processing guide. *Nature Neuroscience Reviews* **7**: 890–901.

Chapter 32
Culham JC and Valyear KF (2006) Human parietal cortex in action. *Curr. Opin.Neurobiol.* **16**:205–212.

Chapter 39
Glickstein M, Schmahmann JD and Caplan D (2006) Thinking about the cerebellum. *Brain* **129**:288–292.

Chapter 50
Cooke SF and Bliss TVP (2006) Plasticity in the human central nervous system. *Brain* **129**:1659–1673.

Chapter 55
Morrison PD and Murray RM,. (2005) Schizophrenia. *Curr.Biol.* **15**: R980–984.

Index

Page numbers in *italics* represent figures, those in **bold** represent tables

LECTURE NOTES

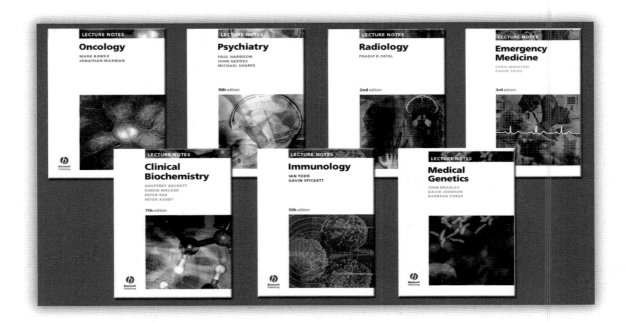

- Concise learning guides for all your subjects
- Focused on what you need to know
- Tried and Trusted

Titles in the LECTURE NOTES series

- Cardiology
- Clinical Anaesthesia
- Clinical Biochemistry
- Clinical Medicine
- Clinical Pharmacology and Therapeutics
- Clinical Skills
- Dermatology
- Diseases of the Ear, Nose and Throat
- Emergency Medicine

- Epidemiology and Public Health Medicine
- General Surgery
- Geriatric Medicine
- Haematology
- Human Physiology
- Immunology
- Infectious Diseases
- Medical Genetics
- Medical Law and Ethics
- Medical Microbiology

- Neurology
- Obstetrics and Gynaecology
- Oncology
- Ophthalmology
- Orthopaedics and Fractures
- Paediatrics
- Psychiatry
- Radiology
- Respiratory Medicine
- Tropical Medicine
- Urology

www.blackwellmedstudent.com Blackwell Publishing